The Nurse

Anaesthetist

The complete Guide

ALEXANDRE CAREWELL

Table of Contents

« *The nurse anaesthetist is not just a technician of drugs and machines; above all, he or she is a vigilant guardian of the patient's sleep and an essential pillar of confidence in the operating theatre.* »

Chapter 1:
INTRODUCTION TO ANAESTHESIA

History and development of anaesthesia

At the heart of medical development, the history of anaesthesia is both fascinating and crucial. It bears witness to mankind's ceaseless quest to relieve pain, transforming countless surgical procedures from unbearable torments into tolerable, even imperceptible interventions.

The origins of anaesthesia go back to antiquity, long before the term itself existed. Early civilisations used herbal and opiate-based potions to put patients to sleep during surgery. The Egyptians, for example, used extracts of opium and mandrake. The Chinese used acupuncture to numb certain parts of the body.

But it was in the 19th century that anaesthesia experienced a real turning point. In 1846, the medical world was shaken when an American dentist named William Morton publicly demonstrated the successful use of ether to put a patient to sleep during a dental extraction in Boston. This demonstration opened the door to the rapid adoption of ether throughout the world.

Ether, however, was not without its drawbacks. It was flammable, had an unpleasant odour and could cause nausea. Other agents, such as chloroform, were introduced shortly afterwards. Chloroform gained popularity after being used to relieve the pain of childbirth by Queen Victoria in 1853. Despite its popularity, it had its own risks, including cardiac toxicity.

In the late 19th and early 20th centuries, significant progress was made with the discovery of cocaine as a local anaesthetic and the introduction of nitrous oxide, which is still used today. At the same time, the development of intubation techniques gave anaesthetists the ability to keep the airway open, changing the landscape for more complex surgery and high-risk patients.

As science progressed, anaesthesia evolved with the advent of barbiturates, benzodiazepines and other intravenous agents. The 20th century saw the rise of electronic patient monitoring, enabling anaesthetists to monitor the heart, blood pressure, oxygenation and other vital parameters in real time, thereby increasing patient safety.

The history of anaesthesia is a reflection of the human capacity to innovate in the face of challenges. It is the story of perseverance, courage and ingenuity. Thanks to these advances, surgeries that were once fatal or impossible have become commonplace, giving new life to millions of people. And as we look to the future, with technologies such as artificial intelligence and personalised anaesthesia, the next pages of this story are sure to be just as, if not more, revolutionary.

Roles and responsibilities
the nurse anaesthetist

The nurse anaesthetist, a central figure in the operating theatre, plays a crucial role in guaranteeing the well-being and safety of patients before, during and after surgery. With specific, in-depth and rigorous training, they are the essential link between the patient, the surgical team and anaesthesiology.

Before the operation :
One of the first roles of the nurse anaesthetist is the pre-anaesthetic assessment. He or she meets the patient, takes a medical history, any allergies, current medication and any other relevant information to anticipate and prevent possible complications. This stage also provides an opportunity to reassure the patient, address any fears and establish a relationship of trust.

He or she is also responsible for preparing the medicines and equipment needed for anaesthesia, ensuring that everything is ready and in order for the operation.

During the intervention :
When the patient is in the operating theatre, the nurse anaesthetist is often the one who administers the anaesthetic, whether general, regional or local. Throughout the operation, they constantly monitor the patient's vital parameters - such as heart rate, blood pressure, oxygen saturation and temperature - and adjust the anaesthetic accordingly to ensure a stable condition.

He also works closely with the surgeon and the medical team, reporting any changes or anomalies and intervening quickly in the event of complications.

After the Intervention :
When the surgery is over, the nurse anaesthetist plays a key role in the patient's recovery. They ensure that the patient wakes up safely, monitor any side effects of the anaesthetic and manage post-operative pain. The anaesthetist is often the first face the patient sees after the operation, offering reassurance and information about the operation.

Additional responsibilities :
In addition to these essential roles, the nurse anaesthetist may also be responsible for training students and new staff, conducting research to improve anaesthetic techniques and participating in hospital committees to ensure high standards of care and safety.

The nurse anaesthetist is a sentinel of patient safety, a pillar of the surgical world, combining technical skills, in-depth medical knowledge and compassion. Their reassuring presence and expertise ensure that, in the complex and ever-changing world of anaesthesia, every patient receives the highest quality of care.

Key features
an efficient nurse anaesthetist

Nurse anaesthetists have a huge responsibility as part of the medical team. To carry out this role competently and ensure the safety and well-being of patients, they must possess a unique combination of professional, interpersonal and emotional qualities. Here are the key characteristics of an effective nurse anaesthetist:

- **Clinical expertise**: At the heart of the profession, a sound knowledge of anaesthetic principles, drugs and techniques is essential. The ability to make rapid decisions based on this expertise is crucial.
- **Attention to detail**: When administering anaesthetics, a small variation in dosage or an omission in patient assessment can have major consequences. A keen eye for detail is therefore essential.
- **Communication skills**: The nurse anaesthetist must be able to communicate effectively with patients, families and the medical team. They must explain

procedures clearly and reassuringly, while being able to listen actively.

Calm under pressure: In the operating theatre, unforeseen situations can arise at any time. The ability to remain calm, think logically and act quickly is fundamental.

Empathy: Understanding and sharing the feelings of others, particularly anxious or frightened patients, helps to build trust and ensure a better patient experience.

Adaptability: Medicine is a constantly evolving field. An effective nurse anaesthetist is ready to adapt to new techniques, technologies and practices to provide the best possible care.

Team spirit: Working in synergy with surgeons, nurses, technicians and other healthcare professionals is essential to ensure the safety and effectiveness of a procedure.

Problem-solving skills: When faced with unexpected challenges or complications, a nurse anaesthetist must be able to think creatively and critically to find solutions.

Professional integrity: Adhering to strict medical ethics, respecting confidentiality and always acting in the patient's best interests are fundamental qualities.

Ongoing commitment to learning: Medicine is advancing by leaps and bounds. An effective nurse anaesthetist constantly seeks out continuing education opportunities to stay at the forefront of their field.

By combining these characteristics, the nurse anaesthetist is not only an expert in anaesthesiology, but also an advocate, educator and essential ally for every patient they encounter. These qualities, when cultivated and honed, make the difference between a competent professional and an exceptional one.

Chapter 2:
FUNDAMENTALS OF ANAESTHESIA

Types of anaesthesia:
general, local, regional

Controlling pain and consciousness during medical procedures is at the heart of anaesthesiology. Depending on the nature of the procedure and the patient's condition, different types of anaesthesia are used. Each has its own advantages, specific applications and considerations. Let's explore these types of anaesthesia together.

- General anaesthesia :
  - **Description**: General anaesthesia places the patient in a state of deep unconsciousness. During this state, the patient feels no pain and has no memory of the procedure.
  - **Method of administration**: It can be administered by inhalation (anaesthetic gases) or by intravenous injection. Often a combination of the two is used.
  - **Use**: Commonly used for major surgery, such as thoracic, abdominal or cardiac operations.
  - **Considerations**: Monitoring of vital parameters is essential. Intubation may be necessary to protect the airway and ensure adequate ventilation.
- Local anaesthesia :
  - **Description**: Local anaesthesia numbs a small specific area of the body, leaving the patient fully conscious.

Method of administration: It is often administered by direct injection into the surgical area.

Use: Typically used for minor procedures such as extracting a tooth, removing a mole or treating a small skin lesion.

Considerations: The patient may feel pressure or movement, but no pain. A slight tingling or burning sensation may be felt during the injection.

Regional anaesthesia :

Description: It numbs a larger area of the body, such as a whole limb or the lower part of the body.

Method of administration :

Plexus nerve block: The anaesthetic is injected close to a nerve plexus, affecting a region of the body such as the arm.

Spinal anaesthesia: The anaesthetic is injected into the cerebrospinal fluid around the spinal cord, numbing the lower part of the body.

Peridural: Similar to spinal anaesthesia, but the anaesthetic is injected into the epidural space around the spinal cord.

Use: Often used for childbirth (epidural), limb surgery or operations on the lower abdomen or pelvis.

Considerations: The patient remains conscious, but the anaesthetised area is insensitive to pain. In some cases, sedatives may be administered to relax the patient.

Each of these types of anaesthesia offers specific advantages depending on the procedure and the patient's needs. The choice depends on many factors, including the nature of the procedure, the patient's state of health, and sometimes the patient's own preference. In all cases, the main aim is to ensure the patient's safety and comfort throughout the operation.

Principles of pharmacology in anaesthesia

Pharmacology is an essential pillar of anaesthesia. Mastery of drugs, their effects and interactions is fundamental to ensuring the safety and efficacy of anaesthesia. Here is an overview of the key principles of pharmacology in anaesthesia:

Pharmacokinetics :

Absorption: How does the drug enter the body? For example, inhaled medicines can be absorbed rapidly by the lungs.

Distribution: Once in the body, how is the drug distributed to the various tissues?

Metabolism: How is the drug transformed or broken down, usually by the liver?

Elimination: How is the drug eliminated from the body, often via the kidneys or breathing?

Pharmacodynamics :

Describes the effect of the drug on the body. How does it work at a cellular or molecular level? For example, some drugs work by blocking ion channels in nerve cells, thereby preventing the transmission of pain.

Inducing agents :

These are the drugs used to induce general anaesthesia. They can be administered intravenously or by inhalation.

Maintenance agents :

Once the patient is under anaesthetic, these drugs maintain the state of unconsciousness. They may include inhaled gases such as sevoflurane or drugs administered by continuous infusion.

Analgesics :

These drugs are used to manage and reduce pain. They include opioids such as fentanyl or morphine and non-opioids such as paracetamol.

Neuromuscular blockers :

Used to induce muscle relaxation, these agents are often used during operations requiring complete immobilisation.

Reversionary agents :

These drugs are used to reverse the effects of other agents, such as neuromuscular blockers.

Vasoactives :

These agents affect vascular tone, blood pressure and cardiac contractility. They are used to support cardiovascular function during anaesthesia.

Sedatives and tranquillisers :

Used to relax and sedate patients before and sometimes after surgery.

Special considerations :

Drug interactions, allergies, genetic variations and medical conditions can all influence the way a patient reacts to a drug. Knowledge and vigilance are essential.

Pharmacology in anaesthesia is a vast and complex field. Each drug has unique characteristics and interacts differently with the body. A thorough understanding of these principles enables the anaesthetist to choose and administer drugs in a way that optimises care while minimising risks.

Monitoring the patient under anaesthesia

Anaesthesia, although routine in many operations, is a delicate procedure that requires close monitoring of the patient. Monitoring during anaesthesia is essential to ensure patient safety, to detect complications early and to guide the anaesthetist's actions. Here is an overview of the key elements of monitoring in anaesthesia:

Cardiovascular monitoring:

- **Electrocardiography (ECG)**: monitoring of the heart's electrical activity, detection of arrhythmias and other cardiac abnormalities.
- **Non-invasive blood pressure (NIBP)**: Regular measurement of blood pressure using a cuff.
- **Invasive Blood Pressure (IBP)**: Continuous measurement of blood pressure via a catheter inserted into an artery, generally used for major surgery or unstable patients.
- **Pulse oximetry**: Measurement of oxygen saturation in the blood using a sensor usually placed on the finger.

Respiratory monitoring:

- **Capnography**: Continuous measurement of exhaled CO_2, essential for assessing ventilation.
- **Tidal Flow and Volume**: Tracks the amount of air inhaled and exhaled with each breath.
- **Inhaled and exhaled gas analysis**: Ensures that the breathing gas mixture is appropriate and that the equipment is operating correctly.

Neurological monitoring:

- **Bispectral Index (BIS):** A measure of the patient's level of consciousness during general anaesthesia.

Neuromuscular monitoring: To monitor the effect of neuromuscular blocking agents and their reversion.

Temperature monitoring:

Monitoring body temperature is crucial, as hypothermia or hyperthermia can have serious consequences during and after surgery.

Diuresis monitoring:

Measuring urine flow can provide information about the patient's renal function and haemodynamic status.

Monitoring the depth of anaesthesia:

Using various devices and techniques, such as BIS, to ensure that the patient is at an appropriate level of anaesthesia.

Gas emboli detectors:

Used in certain surgeries with a high risk of gas embolism.

Haemostatic monitoring:

During surgery with a high risk of bleeding, real-time monitoring of blood coagulation can be crucial.

Alarms and Alerts:

All monitors are equipped with alarms to notify the medical team of any parameter that falls outside normal limits.

Accuracy and speed are essential when monitoring a patient undergoing anaesthesia. Anaesthetists must be trained not only to interpret the data provided by these monitors, but also to respond quickly and appropriately to any anomalies detected. Modern technology has greatly improved patient safety during anaesthesia, but it is the vigilance and expertise of the anaesthetist that really lies at the heart of safe and effective care.

Chapter 3:
THE PRE-OPERATORY

Pre-anaesthetic assessment of the patient

• Case history

History-taking is a fundamental part of medicine. It is the process by which the healthcare professional gathers information about the patient, asking questions about their medical history, current symptoms, lifestyle, habits and other relevant aspects of their health. In the context of anaesthesia, a carefully conducted history is essential to anticipate and prevent potential complications.

Demographic information:
Name, age, sex, weight, height and contact details. This basic information can influence decisions about anaesthesia.

Medical history:
Chronic illnesses (diabetes, hypertension, asthma, heart, kidney or liver disease, etc.).
Surgical history, in particular previous experience with anaesthesia.
History of allergies, including reactions to medication.
Medicines currently being taken, including doses, over-the-counter medicines and food supplements.

History of Anaesthesia:
Previous complications linked to anaesthesia, such as malignant hyperthermia, allergic reactions or other adverse effects.

- Family experience of anaesthesia, as certain complications may have a genetic predisposition.
- Habits and Lifestyle:
  - Consumption of alcohol, tobacco or drugs.
  - Physical activity and level of fitness.
  - Food and diet.
- Current symptoms:
  - In the context of surgery, it is important to understand the patient's current symptoms, the reason for the operation and the duration of the symptoms.
- Clinical examination:
  - Assessment of general condition, cardiac and pulmonary auscultation, examination of the oral cavity to assess ease of intubation.
- Social and family history:
  - Family history of illnesses or medical complications, context of the patient's life (family support, professional environment, etc.).
- Questions specific to anaesthesia:
  - Last meal eaten (to assess the risk of aspiration).
  - Dental problems (risk during intubation).
  - History of sleep apnea or other sleep disorders.
- Patient Concerns and Questions:
  - It is crucial to address any concerns or questions the patient may have about the anaesthetic or the procedure itself.

The history is a crucial stage in establishing a relationship of trust between the patient and the anaesthetist. It is also a key moment for gathering vital information that will guide clinical decisions. In anaesthesia, a careful history can make the difference between a successful operation and potentially serious complications.

• Clinical examination

The clinical examination is an essential stage in the diagnostic process, generally following the history-taking. It is during this examination that the healthcare professional assesses the patient in a methodical and systematic way, using all the senses, often aided by specific instruments, to identify the objective signs of a pathology or condition. For a nurse anaesthetist or anaesthetist, this examination is crucial for assessing the patient's condition before an operation and anticipating any possible challenges or complications.

General review:
> General appearance: posture, nutritional state, level of consciousness.
>
> Vital signs: temperature, pulse, blood pressure, respiratory rate and oxygen saturation.

Examination of the head and neck:
> **Eyes**: pupils, conjunctivae.
>
> **Ears**: external assessment, otoscopy if necessary.
>
> **Mouth**: assessment of dental hygiene, dental mobility (risk during intubation), opening of the mouth, tongue and palate. Visualisation of the oropharynx to anticipate the difficulty of intubation.
>
> **Neck**: mobility, presence of masses, palpation of the trachea, assessment of landmarks for possible cricothyrotomy.

Cardiovascular examination:
> Auscultation of the heart to detect murmurs, irregular rhythms or other abnormalities.
>
> Palpation of peripheral   pulses.

Lung examination:
> Inspection: symmetry, use of accessory muscles.

28

    Palpation: look for crepitations.

    Percussion: assessment of areas of hypo- or hyper-resonance.

    Auscultation: listening to the respiratory sounds, looking for rales, sibilants or other abnormalities.

Abdominal examination:

    Inspection: shape, movements with breathing.

    Auscultation: bowel sounds.

    Palpation: pain, masses, enlarged organs.

    Percussion: assessment of the size of the liver and spleen, and presence of fluid.

Neurological examination:

    Assessment of awareness, orientation and memory.

    Tests of reflexes, strength, sensation and coordination.

    Assessment of cranial nerves.

Musculoskeletal examination:

    Assessment of mobility and strength, and search for deformities or arthritis.

Skin   examination:

    Check for rashes, bruises, sores or other lesions. Assess hydration.

Specific examination for anaesthesia:

    Assessment of the spinal column for possible spinal anaesthesia or epidural.

    Assessment of veins for a potential intravenous access route.

The clinical examination, complementing the history, provides a complete picture of the patient's condition. For an anaesthetist, it enables difficulties to be anticipated, the anaesthetic plan to be adjusted and the patient's safety and well-being to be guaranteed before, during and after surgery.

• Further investigations

After the medical history and clinical examination, further investigations play a key role in preparing a patient for an operation requiring anaesthesia. These investigations provide objective data on the patient's state of health, enabling a more thorough assessment of the risks and optimal planning of the anaesthetic.

Blood analysis:

Blood count (CBC): To assess anaemia, infection or other hematology disorders.

Liver and kidney   tests: These give an indication of the functioning of the liver and kidneys, which are essential for metabolising and eliminating anaesthetic drugs.

Prothrombin time (PT) and activated partial thromboplastin   time (APTT): To assess coagulation.

Blood sugar: Particularly in diabetic patients.

Electrolytes: Sodium, potassium, chlorine, bicarbonate, to assess imbalances that could influence the response to anaesthesia.

Electrocardiogram (ECG):

Essential for patients with a history of heart disease or certain risk factors. ECG may reveal arrhythmias, ischaemia or other cardiac abnormalities.

Chest X-ray:

May be requested in the event of respiratory symptoms, smoking, or for major operations.

Spirometry:

An assessment of lung function, particularly in patients with a history of lung disease such as asthma or COPD.

Echocardiography:

For patients with heart murmurs, heart failure or other cardiac pathologies, to assess the function and structure of the heart.

Allergy tests:

If the patient has a history of allergies, specific tests can be carried out to identify the precise agents to which the patient is allergic.

Other images:

Depending on the nature of the procedure and the patient's history, other forms of imaging such as CT scan, MRI or angiography may be required.

Specialist consultations:

Depending on the patient's co-morbidities, consultations with other specialists (cardiologist, pulmonologist, nephrologist, etc.) may be required to assess and optimise the patient's condition prior to surgery.

Additional investigations are not systematically requested for every patient, but are decided on the basis of the patient's specific needs and the nature of the operation. The main objective is to ensure patient safety by minimising the risks associated with anaesthesia and the surgery itself.

Mental preparation and emotional state of the patient

Preparing for surgery involves more than just physical assessment and tests. The mental and emotional aspect is just as crucial. Patients facing surgery may experience a variety of emotions, including anxiety, fear or even depression. Addressing and managing these emotional aspects can greatly influence the patient's experience and, in some cases, even their post-operative results.

Assessment of Anxiety:

- Recognise the signs of anxiety, such as nervousness, sleep problems or physical symptoms like palpitations.
- Use standardised assessment tools, such as the Amsterdam Preoperative Anxiety Questionnaire, to quantify anxiety.

Effective communication:

- Provide clear, comprehensible information about the procedure, anaesthesia, risks and recovery process.
- Allow the patient time to ask questions and ensure full answers.

Relaxation techniques:

- Encourage deep breathing, visualisation or meditation to help reduce anxiety.
- In some cases, pre-operative training in these techniques may be offered.

Psychotherapeutic support:

- For particularly anxious patients, consider consulting a psychologist or psychotherapist.
- Interventions such as cognitive behavioural therapy can be beneficial.

Involvement of family and friends:

- Involving the patient's family or close friends in the preparation process can provide additional emotional support.

Preparing for post-operative pain:

- Inform the patient about possible post-operative pain and strategies for managing it.
- Reassurance about effective pain management.

Pharmacological support:

- For some patients, medication such as anxiolytics may be prescribed before the operation.

Workshops and support groups:
　　Some hospitals offer workshops or support groups for patients undergoing surgery, enabling them to share their concerns and learn from the experiences of others.

Mental and emotional preparation is essential to ensure that the patient approaches the operation in the best possible conditions. Such preparation can not only improve the patient's experience but also positively influence their recovery and post-operative results.

Anticipating clinical challenges

In the field of anaesthesia, nurse anaesthetists are faced with a wide range of clinical challenges, which they must anticipate and manage competently. These challenges can vary depending on the type of surgery, the patient's state of health and many other factors. Anticipating them can help minimise risks and ensure patient safety.

Difficult anatomy:
　　Identify patients with difficult airways or complex vascular anatomy in advance to facilitate intubation and catheterisation.
　　Use tools such as the Mallampati classification to assess the risk of difficult intubation.
Comorbidities:
　　Recognise patients with significant co-morbidities (heart, lung, kidney disease, etc.) that could affect their response to anaesthesia or increase the risk of complications.

Allergic reactions:

> Knowing the patient's allergy history so as to avoid drugs or products that could cause a reaction.

Pain management:

> Anticipate the patient's analgesic needs, particularly for procedures known to cause significant post-operative pain.

Potential complications:

> Be prepared for complications such as aspiration, hypoxia, hypotension or other adverse events.

Equipment and Technology:

> Ensuring that the necessary equipment is available and working properly, and preparing for any malfunctions.

Drug interactions:

> Be aware of the medicines the patient is taking regularly and anticipate any possible interaction with anaesthetic drugs.

Management of paediatric and elderly patients:

> Children and the elderly present unique challenges when it comes to anaesthesia. Specific training and preparation is essential for these populations.

Physiological changes during surgery:

> Anticipate possible fluctuations in body temperature, fluid levels and electrolyte balance during the operation.

Communication:

Ensuring clear communication with the surgical team, the patient and the family to anticipate and resolve problems quickly.

Anticipating clinical challenges requires a combination of training, experience and vigilance. By preparing in advance, nurse anaesthetists can ensure that the patient receives the best possible care while minimising the risks associated with anaesthesia and surgery.

Chapter 4:
IN THE OPERATING ROOM

Induction techniques
and anaesthetic maintenance

Anaesthetic induction is the process by which a patient moves from the conscious to the anaesthetised state, while maintenance refers to the period during which the patient remains under anaesthesia. Induction and maintenance techniques are crucial to ensuring safe and painless surgery.

Intravenous induction:

- **Agents used**: Propofol, thiopental, etomidate, ketamine.
- Used for their rapid action, they are administered intravenously, causing rapid loss of consciousness.

Inhalation induction:

- **Agents used**: Sevoflurane, desflurane, isoflurane.
- Often used in children or when intravenous access is difficult. The patient breathes the anaesthetic gas through a mask.

Opiates:

- **Agents used**: Fentanyl, remifentanil, morphine, sufentanil.
- Help with pain management and can be used during induction and maintenance to enhance the anaesthetic effect.

Neuromuscular blocking agents:

- **Agents used**: Rocuronium, succinylcholine, atracurium.

Used to facilitate intubation and induce muscle relaxation during surgery.

Anaesthetic maintenance:

Can be performed using intravenous agents such as propofol in continuous infusion or inhaled agents such as sevoflurane or desflurane.

Balanced Anaesthesia Techniques:

Combine several agents, such as opiates, intravenous agents and inhaled agents, to optimise anaesthesia while minimising side effects.

Monitoring:

Essential during induction and maintenance to monitor depth of anaesthesia, cardiovascular function, pulmonary function and other critical parameters.

Ventilation:

Once the patient is under anaesthetic, ventilation is generally provided by a respirator, depending on the needs of the patient and the surgery.

Regional Techniques:

Can be used as a complement to general anaesthesia or as the main technique. Examples: nerve blocks, epidurals, spinal anaesthesia.

Wake up:

After surgery, the anaesthetic agents are stopped or reversed, and the patient is carefully monitored until he or she recovers consciousness and adequate respiratory function.

Anaesthetic induction and maintenance techniques require expertise and a thorough understanding of pharmacology, physiology and anaesthetic equipment. The main aim is to ensure that the patient remains comfortable, pain-free and safe throughout the surgical procedure.

Airway management

Airway management is one of the most fundamental and critical skills for a nurse anaesthetist. Adequate mastery of this skill is essential to ensure adequate ventilation and oxygenation of the patient during anaesthesia. Let's approach this in a fluid way, detailing the key elements:

Evaluation of airways:
>
> The importance of this stage cannot be underestimated. It includes a physical examination (such as the Mallampati classification, thyromental distance, neck mobility), the patient's medical history and, if necessary, imaging tests.

Positioning:
>
> The position of the head and neck can greatly influence the ease of intubation. The so-called "rose scent" position - alignment of the ears with the sternum using cushions - is frequently used.

Oxygenation Pre-oxygenation:
>
> Before any attempt at intubation, it i s advisable to pre-oxygenate the patient to increase oxygen reserves, which provides a longer delay in the event of intubation difficulties.

Intubation techniques:
>
> Orotracheal intubation is the most common, but nasotracheal intubation may be necessary for some surgeries. The use of video-laryngoscopes can facilitate visualisation of the airway.

Mask ventilation:
>
> In certain situations, it may be necessary to ventilate the patient using a face mask before

intubation, or if intubation is delayed or impossible.

Supraglottic devices:
These devices, such as the laryngeal mask, can be used as an alternative to tracheal intubation or as a rescue tool when intubation is difficult.

Difficult air routes:
If intubation fails, having a clear plan and specific devices (such as fibre-optic laryngoscopes) is crucial. Regular training on mannequins and workshops can help prepare for these situations.

Extubation:
Safe removal of the intubation tube at the end of surgery is as crucial as its insertion. We need to ensure that the patient is fully awake, has intact reflexes and can protect his or her airway.

Complications:
Being aware of and prepared for potential complications such as aspiration, airway trauma or bronchospasm is essential.

Ongoing training:
With the advent of new technologies and techniques, ongoing training and simulations of emergency scenarios are essential.

Airway management is a delicate dance between science and art, requiring perfect synchronisation of skill, know-how and presence of mind. In the hands of a skilled nurse anaesthetist, this dance ensures safe and effective surgery.

Advanced monitoring and its importance

Advanced monitoring in the operating theatre and recovery room transcends standard methods, offering a more in-depth assessment of patient physiology. In a medical context where every second counts, these advanced tools provide clinicians with a valuable window into their patients' condition, enabling them to anticipate and respond rapidly to dynamic changes that may occur.

- Hemodynamic monitoring:
    - **Transoesophageal echocardiography (TEE)**: Provides real-time images of the heart, allowing assessment of cardiac function, ventricular volumes, and detection of possible valvular or pericardial pathology.
    - **Impedance Cardiometry**: Uses electrical currents to estimate cardiac output, preload and other haemodynamic parameters.
    - **Analysis of Blood Pressure Variability**: An indirect measure of preload, vascular reactivity and baroreflex reactivity.
- Neurological monitoring:
    - **Bispectral Index (BIS):** A tool for assessing the depth of anaesthesia by analysing brain waves, in order to avoid anaesthesia that is too deep or too light.
    - **Near-Infrared Spectroscopy (NIRS)**: measures oxygen saturation in the brain, useful for monitoring cerebral perfusion during major cardiovascular or neurosurgical procedures.
- Tissue Perfusion Monitoring:
    - **Lactate monitoring**: An indirect indicator of tissue perfusion, with high levels suggesting hypoperfusion or ischaemia.
    - **Capnography**: A measurement of exhaled CO_2, which is crucial for monitoring ventilation,

but also tissue perfusion in certain circumstances.

Respiratory function monitoring:

- **Electrical Impedance Tomography**: A non-invasive technique for visualising lung volume distribution in real time. It can help optimise ventilation strategy in patients with lung damage.

Importance of Advanced Monitoring:

- **Anticipation**: Enables clinicians to anticipate complications before they become critical.
- **Individualised care**: Promotes personalised care, adapting interventions to the patient's specific needs.
- **Optimising Results**: Reduces morbidity and mortality by enabling faster, more accurate interventions.
- **Research and Education**: Provides a basis for clinical research and education, offering real-time learning opportunities.

In the complex world of anaesthesia and perioperative care, advanced monitoring is a lifeline, an interface between the clinician and the patient's essential physiological systems. Just as a navigator uses instruments to safely navigate unknown waters, the nurse anaesthetist relies on these tools to safely guide the patient through the challenges of surgery and anaesthesia.

Management intraoperative complications

Intraoperative complications are among the most feared challenges in anaesthesiology. The speed and accuracy of the response can make the difference between a transient event with no consequences and a catastrophic outcome.

Understanding and mastering the management of these complications is essential for the nurse anaesthetist.

Hypoxaemia and hypoventilation:
Possible causes: obstruction or displacement of the endotracheal tube, bronchospasm, pneumothorax, aspiration.

Interventions: Ensure adequate oxygenation, check tube position, administer bronchodilators, consider endotracheal suctioning, or chest drainage if pneumothorax is suspected.

Hypotension:
Possible causes: haemorrhage, anaphylactic reaction, cardiogenic reaction, sepsis, anaesthetic depression.

Interventions: Administration of fluids, vasopressors, antihistamines, corticosteroids, inotropic support and identification and correction of the underlying cause.

Hypertension:
Possible causes: hypercarbia, surgical retraction, bladder hypertrophy, hyperthermia, systemic inflammatory response syndrome.

Interventions : Antihypertensives, further anaesthesia, temperature management and treatment of the underlying cause.

Cardiac dysrhythmias:
Possible causes: Ischaemia, electrolyte imbalance, hypoxia, hypercarbia.

Interventions: Antiarrhythmics, oxygenation, correction of electrolyte imbalances, cardioversion if necessary.

Increase in end-expiratory CO2:
Possible causes: hypoventilation, pulmonary embolism, faulty anaesthetic circuit.

Interventions: Check ventilation, assess anaesthetic circuit, consider cardiac ultrasound for embolism.

Hypothermia:

Possible causes: Blood transfusion, heat loss in the operating theatre, drug reaction.

Interventions: heated blankets, heated liquids, limiting skin exposure.

Awakening during anaesthesia:

Possible causes: Inadequate dosage of anaesthetic agents, equipment malfunction.

Interventions: Administering additional anaesthetic agents, reassuring the patient after the operation.

Mechanical complications:

Possible causes: Burns from electric scalpel plates, explosions from flammable gas mixtures, position-related injuries.

Interventions: Regularly checking equipment and patient position, following strict safety protocols.

The key to managing intraoperative complications lies in prevention, early detection and rapid intervention. The nurse anaesthetist must work closely with the surgeon and surgical team, anticipating potential problems and being well prepared with the knowledge and skills to deal with them. In this dynamic environment, clear communication and team coordination are essential to ensure patient safety.

Chapter 5:
AFTER THE OPERATION

Post-anaesthetic monitoring

The period immediately following an anaesthetic, often referred to as the recovery phase, is critical. During this period, the patient is in transition between the state of deep anaesthesia and the return to basal normality. Post-anaesthetic monitoring is essential to ensure patient safety and comfort.

- Surveillance site:
  - **Recovery Room or Post Anaesthetic Care Unit (PACU)**: This is where the majority of patients are brought after surgery for close monitoring by specialist staff.
- Vital functions:
  - **Heart Rate and Rhythm**: Any changes should be noted and assessed.
  - **Blood pressure**: Variations may indicate problems such as bleeding or drug reactions.
  - **Oxygen saturation**: Crucial for detecting any residual hypoxia.
  - **Respiratory rate**: To ensure that the patient is breathing adequately after anaesthesia.
- Neurological condition:
  - **Level of Consciousness**: Is the patient returning to a basal state? Are there any signs of waking during anaesthesia or of excessive drowsiness?
  - **Orientation**: Is he able to answer basic questions about the place, the date and his identity?

Movement of the extremities: Make sure there are no post-operative neurological deficits.

Pain management:

Regularly assess the patient's pain using standardised scales and administer analgesics as required.

Management of post-operative nausea and vomiting (PONV):

Identify patients at risk, administer prophylactic or therapeutic antiemetics if necessary.

Thermal management:

Monitor body temperature. Use warm blankets or other means to warm hypothermic patients.

Inspection of surgical sites:

Watch for bleeding, bruising or any other abnormal signs.

Assessment of Urinary and Gastrointestinal Function:

Monitor urine output and the presence of gas or Feces if relevant to the procedure.

Assessment of Respiratory Function:

Make sure the patient can cough and breathe deeply. Watch for congestion or other signs of respiratory complications.

Documentation:

Record all medicines administered, vital signs, assessments and interventions in the patient record.

Exit criteria:

Use standardised criteria, such as the Aldrete score, to determine when a patient is ready to leave the PACU.

Post-anaesthetic monitoring is a crucial phase in the perioperative process, during which complications can arise rapidly. Rigorous observation, rapid intervention and effective communication are essential to ensure the patient's safety and well-being during this transitional period.

Post-operative pain management

Post-operative pain is one of the main concerns of patients after surgery. Adequate pain management is not only humane, it also facilitates recovery, reduces complications and improves patient satisfaction. Here is a fluid description of postoperative pain management.

After surgery, pain is a natural bodily reaction, but that doesn't mean it has to be endured in silence. Effective management of postoperative pain is a symphony in which several players - doctors, anaesthetists, nurses and even the patient - play an essential role.

Pain assessment:
Before pain can be treated, it is essential to measure it. The use of pain scales, such as the visual analogue scale (VAS) or the numerical scale, offers a standardised method of assessing pain intensity. This assessment should be regular and consistent, taking into account both the intensity and the nature of the pain.

Multimodal approach:
The idea behind multimodal management is to use several types of medication and techniques to reduce pain, thereby reducing the dose of each agent and, consequently, minimising side effects.

Analgesics:
  Non-opioid analgesics: Paracetamol and non-steroidal anti-inflammatory drugs (NSAIDs) such as ibuprofen can be used to treat mild to moderate pain.

Opiates: Drugs such as morphine, fentanyl or oxycodone are powerful and effective, but should be used with caution due to their potential side effects.

Local anaesthetics: Administered directly to the surgical site or via regional techniques such as nerve blocks, they can offer effective relief without the systemic effects of opiates.

Complementary Techniques:
Methods such as cryotherapy, transcutaneous electrical nerve stimulation (TENS) or even certain complementary therapies, such as acupuncture, can be effective.

Non-medication strategies:
Relaxation techniques, distraction, music therapy or cognitive behavioural therapies can play a complementary role in pain management.

Patient education:
An informed patient is a partner in treatment. It is vital to explain the options available, pain expectations and potential side-effects. The goal is not always total absence of pain, but manageable pain that allows functional recovery.

Monitoring side effects:
Pain and its treatment can have consequences. Constipation, nausea, itching or respiratory depression are possible side effects, especially with opioids. Their early recognition and management are just as crucial as the treatment of the pain itself.

Postoperative pain management is a delicate balance between effective pain relief and minimising side effects. It's a delicate dance that every healthcare professional must learn to perfect, always with the patient's well-being at the heart of every decision.

Common post-anaesthetic complications and their management

Post-anaesthetic complications can vary from patient to patient depending on their state of health, the type of surgery and the anaesthetic used. Although the majority of anaesthesias are uneventful, it is crucial for healthcare professionals to be prepared to recognise and manage potential complications. Here is an exploration of these complications and strategies for dealing with them.

1. Postoperative Nausea and Vomiting (PONV):
   Description: PONV can occur in up to 30% of patients, especially after certain types of surgery, such as ear, nose or throat surgery.
   Management: Administration of antiemetics such as ondansetron, metoclopramide or dexamethasone. Proactive prevention is also recommended for high-risk patients.
2. Hypoxaemia (low level of oxygen in the blood):
   Presentation: Cyanosis, confusion and low oxygen saturation are common signs.
   Management: administer oxygen, assess the airway and look for underlying causes such as atelectasis or pulmonary oedema.
3. Respiratory depression:
   Presentation: Low respiratory rate, difficulty waking up, reduced oxygen saturation.
   Management: Stimulation of the patient, checking the airway, administration of oxygen. In severe cases, naloxone may be used to reverse the effects of opioids.
4. Uncontrolled pain:
   Presentation: Severe pain, despite standard analgesic medication.

Management: Pain reassessment, adjustment of analgesic medication, use of multimodal approaches.

5. Hypothermia or hyperthermia:

Presentation: Abnormally low or high body temperature after surgery.

Management: For hypothermia, warm the patient with warming blankets. For hyperthermia, look for causes such as neuroleptic malignant syndrome or malignant hyperthermia, and treat accordingly.

6. Bradycardia or tachycardia:

Presentation: Abnormally low or high heart rate.

Management: Identification and treatment of the underlying cause. Atropine for bradycardia or anti-arrhythmic agents for tachycardia, as appropriate.

7. Allergic reactions:

Presentation: Skin rashes, itching, swelling, breathing difficulties.

Management: Stop the suspected drug, administer antihistamine, corticosteroid therapy or adrenaline, depending on the severity.

8. Urinary retention:

Presentation: Inability to urinate after surgery, abdominal discomfort.

Management: Assessment of post-micturition residual, catheterisation if necessary.

9. Postoperative confusion or delirium:

Presentation: Disorientation, agitation, hallucinations.

Management: Ensuring the patient's safety, reassessing medication, hydration and sometimes administration of antipsychotics.

The key to managing post-anaesthetic complications is careful monitoring, early recognition of problems and prompt intervention. Each complication has its own nuances, but with the right training and a well-coordinated team, most can be managed effectively to ensure patient safety and comfort.

Chapter 6:
SPECIAL TECHNIQUES IN ANAESTHESIA

Paediatric anaesthesia : challenges and particularities

Paediatric anaesthesia is a delicate speciality that requires not only an in-depth knowledge of the physiological particularities of children, but also sensitivity to their psychological and emotional needs. Administering anaesthesia to a child is not simply a question of 'miniaturising' adult practice. Here is a fluid exploration of the challenges and particularities that characterise paediatric anaesthesia.

The first thing you notice about a child is its small size, but this smallness conceals immense complexity. Children's physiological systems are constantly evolving, which makes paediatrics unique and stimulating.

1. Physiological challenges:

Respiratory system: Children's airways are proportionately narrower, making intubation and mechanical ventilation more delicate. In addition, children have a higher oxygen consumption, making them more susceptible to hypoxia.

Cardiovascular system: Children have a more limited cardiac capacity to compensate for blood loss, making close monitoring during surgery crucial.

Drug metabolism: The way in which children metabolise drugs differs from that of adults. Doses often need to be adjusted according to weight or body surface area, rather than simply reduced proportionally.

2. Psychological challenges:

    Pre-operative anxiety: Fear of the unknown is common in children. It is crucial to reassure them, sometimes with the help of pre-anaesthetic drugs, but also using non-medicinal techniques such as play or distraction.

    Separation from parents: This separation can be traumatic. Many institutions allow parents to accompany their child to the operating theatre to reduce anxiety.

3. Technical features:

    Respiratory tract: Equipment to secure paediatric airways must be specific to the size of the child, from premature babies to adolescents.

    Vascular access: Children's veins are smaller, making catheter insertion more delicate.

4. Specific pathologies:

Many conditions, such as certain congenital heart diseases or malformations, are specific to the paediatric population. A thorough understanding of these conditions is essential for the paediatric anaesthetist.

5. Communication:

Communicating with a child requires a different approach to that of an adult. Paediatric anaesthetists must be able to explain procedures in a way that is understandable and reassuring for the child.

Paediatric anaesthesia is a delicate balance between science and art. Every child is unique, with his or her own needs and challenges. But with the right training, a patient approach and a deep understanding of the particularities of paediatrics, the paediatric anaesthetist is able to provide optimal care to this particularly vulnerable population.

Anaesthesia for obstetric surgery

Obstetric surgery, in particular caesarean section, is one of the most common surgical procedures in the world. The anaesthetic management of these procedures is unique due to the physiological changes associated with pregnancy, the presence of two patients (mother and foetus) and the particular challenges associated with the urgency of certain situations. Here is a fluid exploration of anaesthesia in obstetrics.

The obstetric operating theatre is a place where every second counts. It's a place where life often begins, but it's also a place where life can quickly be put at risk without appropriate care.

1. Physiological changes during pregnancy:
   Respiratory system: Due to the increase in uterine volume, the diaphragm is pushed upwards, reducing functional residual capacity. This makes pregnant women more vulnerable to hypoxia.
   Cardiovascular system: Blood volume increases during pregnancy, modifying the mother's haemodynamic response.
   Gastrointestinal: Increased progesterone levels slow gastric emptying, increasing the risk of aspiration.

2. Types of Anaesthesia for Obstetric Surgery:
   Peridural: This regional anaesthetic is commonly used for vaginal deliveries and caesarean sections. It has the advantage of preserving the mother's consciousness while providing effective analgesia.
   Spinal anaesthesia: A rapid and effective technique, often used for caesarean sections. It involves injecting local anaesthetic into the cerebrospinal fluid.
   General anaesthesia: Although less common for scheduled caesarean sections, it may be necessary in

an emergency or if regional anaesthesia is not possible.

3. Airway Management:
Intubation can be more difficult in pregnant women due to anatomical and physiological changes. Careful preparation is essential to minimise the risks.

4. Foetal monitoring:
As well as monitoring the mother, it is crucial to monitor the well-being of the foetus. The foetal heart rate is a valuable indicator of the state of the foetus during surgery.

5. Potential Complications:
- **Mendelson's syndrome: This is** aspiration pneumonitis due to inhalation of acidic gastric contents. Prevention is key, using antacids and ensuring prompt and effective intubation if necessary.
- **Local Anaesthetic Toxicity**: Overdose may result in neurological or cardiovascular symptoms.

6. Postoperative pain:
Post-operative pain management is essential to promote recovery and breastfeeding. Analgesics, combined with regional anaesthesia, can be used.

7. Emergency anaesthesia:
In the event of acute foetal distress or uterine rupture, an emergency caesarean section may be necessary. The anaesthetist must be prepared to act quickly while ensuring the safety of both mother and baby.

Obstetric anaesthesia is a delicate balancing act, requiring meticulous care for both mother and foetus. The ability to react quickly to changes while guaranteeing the safety of both patients makes this speciality unique and essential.

Anaesthesia in emergency situations and traumatology

Emergencies and trauma represent one of the most tense and unpredictable areas of medicine. The anaesthetist plays a crucial role in stabilising, assessing and preparing traumatised or seriously ill patients for emergency surgery. In these circumstances, every decision counts and every second can make a difference.

The whistle of monitors, the clatter of instruments, the rapid exchange of orders between team members: a trauma room in action is the scene of an orchestrated symphony in which the anaesthetist is often the conductor.

1. Initial Assessment and Stabilisation:
   Injury triage: Quickly identifying patients who require immediate intervention is vital. Triage systems, such as the Trauma Score, can help.
   Airway: Ensuring a safe airway is a priority. This may require emergency intubation, sometimes in less than ideal conditions.
   Haemodynamics: Stabilisation of blood pressure and correction of haemodynamic drifts are essential. Fluids, blood transfusions and vasopressor drugs may be necessary.
2. Assessment of the severity of the trauma:
   Primary examination: Rapid identification of vital problems, often following the ABCDE sequence (Airway, Breathing, Circulation, Disability, Exposure).
   Secondary examination: A more detailed assessment to identify other potential injuries.
3. Preparing for anaesthesia:
   Anticipating Difficulties: Due to injuries or concomitant conditions, anaesthesia can present challenges, such as difficult airways or haemodynamic instability.

54

Choice of Anaesthetic Agents: In the context of trauma, certain agents may be preferred because of their haemodynamic profiles or side effects.

4. Airway Management in Trauma:

Risks: Injuries to the head, neck or face can complicate intubation.

Rapid Intubation Techniques: These techniques aim to secure the airway quickly while minimising the risk of aspiration or other complications.

5. Monitoring in Emergency Situations:

Standard monitoring: This includes blood pressure, ECG, oxygen saturation and, in some cases, capnography.

Advanced Monitoring: Depending on the situation, this may include invasive blood pressure measurement, anaesthetic depth monitoring or continuous haemoglobin monitoring.

6. Complications and Special Challenges:

Neck injuries: The risk of spinal cord injury must be taken into account when handling the neck.

Traumatic shock: This is a complex response to severe blood loss which may require careful management of fluids, vasoactive agents and transfusions.

Thoracic and abdominal injuries: These injuries can influence the choice and management of anaesthesia.

7. Post anaesthesia and intensive care:

After surgery, many trauma patients require monitoring in an intensive care unit. The anaesthetist plays a role in the transition and recommendation of post-operative management.

Anaesthesia in emergency and trauma situations is a challenge. It demands speed, precision and flexibility. Anaesthetists working in this field are often faced with difficult decisions, but their expertise is essential to optimise outcomes for seriously injured or ill patients.

Chapter 7:
SIMULATION IN ANAESTHESIA

The importance of simulation in training

The world is changing at breakneck speed, and with it the demands of modern professions. Whether in aeronautics, medicine or even education, simulation has become a cornerstone of training. It represents a bridge between academic theory and real-life practice, allowing learners to experiment, make mistakes and learn in a controlled environment.

Imagine a young airline pilot, hands clammy, heart pounding, preparing to land for the first time in dense fog. Or a novice surgeon about to perform a delicate procedure. Thanks to simulation, these stressful scenarios can be safely experienced before they are encountered in real life.

1. Experiential learning:
Humans learn best through experience. Simulation offers a unique opportunity to 'do' rather than simply 'listen' or 'read'. It actively involves the learner, enhancing retention and understanding.

2. Risk-free environment:
One of the greatest strengths of simulation is that it allows learners to make mistakes without any real consequences. It is in these moments of error that the most valuable lessons are often found.

3. Standardisation of training:
Simulation ensures that every learner is exposed to the same scenarios or situations, guaranteeing a consistent training experience.

4. Immediate feedback:
With modern technology, simulations can offer real-time feedback, allowing learners to adjust their actions and understand their mistakes on the spot.

5. Preparing for Rare Scenarios:
In professions such as medicine, certain critical events are rare. Simulation allows professionals to train for these unlikely events, ensuring that they are ready on the day they occur.

6. Development of non-technical skills:
As well as technical skills, simulation can help develop communication, decision-making and teamwork skills, which are often crucial in emergency situations.

7. Assessment and validation of skills:
Modern simulators offer detailed metrics that can be used to assess a learner's competence and progress.

8. Continuous Improvement:
By using simulation to test new procedures or equipment, institutions can ensure that they are optimal before deploying them in real-life situations.

9. Cost reduction:
Although the implementation of simulations may require an initial investment, it can reduce costs in the long term by lowering the error rate, optimising training and reducing training time.

10. Adaptability:
With advances in technology, simulations can be adapted for a multitude of scenarios, skills and levels of complexity, ensuring relevant training at all levels.

In a constantly changing world, simulation is more than a tool: it's a necessity. It prepares professionals to meet tomorrow's challenges with skill and confidence, ensuring that when they are confronted with real-life situations, they are not doing so for the first time.

Common scenarios and how to use them effectively

Scenario-based simulation is a powerful training and assessment method. It reproduces specific situations or challenges that professionals might encounter in the real world. The key to the success of this method lies in creating well-designed scenarios and using them effectively. Let's take a look at some common scenarios and tips on how to make the most of them.

Current scenarios:

Medical Emergency Scenarios: These reproduce situations such as cardiac arrest, a severe allergic reaction or haemorrhage. They enable healthcare professionals to practise emergency procedures.

Difficult Communication Scenarios: These scenarios involve situations where it is necessary to communicate difficult news to a patient or their family, manage an aggressive patient or work as part of a team during a crisis.

Crisis Management Scenarios: These can be applied to many areas, from managing an aviation emergency to responding to a major industrial incident.

Technical scenarios: These focus on mastering specific skills, such as handling new equipment.

Decision-Making Scenarios: These scenarios focus on rapidly assessing complex situations and making decisions accordingly.

How to use them effectively:

Define clear objectives: Before designing or choosing a scenario, it is essential to define what you want participants to learn or practise.

Realism: The more realistic the scenario, the more immersive it is, which encourages learning. Use high-tech props, actors or simulators if possible.

- **Pre-Scenario Briefing**: Before you start, clearly explain the context, objectives and expectations. This will help participants to engage fully.
- **Post-Script Debrief**: This is one of the most crucial stages. After the script, discuss what went well, what could have been done differently and what lessons can be learned.
- **Evaluation**: Provide constructive feedback. Use evaluation grids to give structured feedback to participants.
- **Flexibility**: Be prepared to adapt the scenario according to the reactions and needs of the participants. Sometimes a scenario can take an unexpected direction, and that's fine.
- **Rehearsal**: As with any skill, regular practice is essential. Organise regular simulation sessions to enable continuous improvement.
- **Updating scenarios**: As technologies, procedures or protocols evolve, your scenarios also need to be updated.
- **Create a Safe Environment**: Make sure participants feel comfortable making mistakes and learning from them.
- **Using technology**: Modern technology offers incredibly realistic simulators, from video feedback systems to robotic mannequins.

Scenario-based simulation is a valuable tool, but its effectiveness depends on the quality of the scenarios and how they are used. With careful preparation, thoughtful implementation and appropriate feedback, they can transform professional training and preparation.

Feedback and lessons learned from simulation

Simulation, like any educational innovation, has had its dazzling successes and its learning moments. By integrating these experiences into the medical landscape and beyond, many lessons have been learned. Let's take a look at some of the lessons learned and the insights they have provided.

1. To err is human, and an opportunity:
A young doctor recounted how, during his first simulation, he had accidentally administered a dose of adrenaline ten times higher than necessary. This mistake, which could have had tragic consequences in real life, became a crucial teaching moment. The simulation revealed that mistakes are not just errors, but also opportunities to learn in a risk-free environment.

2. Communication is the Key:
In a simulated plane crash rescue scenario, a team found that despite their individual skills, their communication was chaotic, leading to delays and duplication of effort. This experience underlined that technical competence alone is not enough; effective communication is essential.

3. Technology does not replace human judgement:
A complex simulation scenario using state-of-the-art robotic mannequins showed a medical team that, although technology can reproduce vital signs and symptoms, it cannot always replicate the subtlety of human responses. It is vital not to rely solely on technology, but also to trust your intuition and clinical judgement.

4. Practice Makes Perfect:
One nurse shared how repeating a particularly difficult scenario had helped her master a skill she previously found daunting. She noted that the ability to practice repeatedly in a simulated environment had boosted her confidence and competence.

5. Debriefing is invaluable:

After a simulated surgical crisis, one surgeon expressed his gratitude for the debriefing session that followed. This was an opportunity for the team to openly discuss the challenges encountered, mistakes made and strategies for improvement. This constructive feedback was considered as valuable, if not more so, than the simulation itself.

6. Flexibility is essential:

In an obstetric emergency scenario, one team realised that, despite meticulous planning, real-life situations can take unexpected turns. The ability to adapt and react quickly to a changing situation is an essential skill that simulation can help to develop.

Simulation, while powerful, is not a panacea. It provides an environment for testing, making mistakes, learning and improving. But the most profound lessons often come from participants' feedback, which shows just how transformative this tool can be when used effectively.

Chapter 8:
COMMUNICATION
IN THE OPERATING ROOM

Effective communication techniques with the surgical team

Communication within the surgical team is a crucial element in ensuring patient safety, smooth surgery and harmonious collaboration between the different team members. Discover some tried and tested techniques for effective communication in the operating theatre:

1. Preoperative briefing:
   - Before any operation, arrange a preoperative meeting to discuss the essential points: surgical plan, anaesthetic requirements, patient history, etc.
   - Make sure every member of the team has a clear understanding of their role.
2. The SBAR Technique (Situation, Background, Assessment, Recommendation):
   - **Situation**: Briefly describe the current problem.
   - **Background**: Give the relevant context or background.
   - **Assessment**: Share your assessment of the situation.
   - **Recommendation**: Suggest an action or ask a question.
3. Using checklists:
   - Checklists, such as the WHO Surgical Safety Checklist, can greatly improve communication and prevent oversights.
4. Assertive communication:
   - Express your needs or concerns clearly, without being aggressive or passive. Mutual respect is the key.

5. Clarification and reformulation:
   If an instruction or piece of information is not clear, ask for clarification. Also rephrase to confirm that you have understood correctly.
6. Non-verbal communication:
   Watch your body language and be aware of that of others. Gestures, facial expressions and tone of voice can often convey as much information as words themselves.
7. Active listening:
   Concentrate on the person speaking, nod, ask questions and avoid interrupting.
8. Use of Technology:
   Wireless communication systems, intercoms or even simple light signals can help to communicate effectively without disrupting the workflow.
9. Constructive feedback:
   After the event, take the time to give and receive feedback. Constructive feedback can help to improve future collaboration.
10. Communication training:
    Encourage the team to take part in specific communication training, particularly in high-pressure situations.
11. Avoid jargon:
    Although the surgical team is familiar with medical jargon, it is always preferable to use clear terms, especially in the presence of less experienced members.
12. Create an environment of trust:
    Foster a culture where every team member feels comfortable asking questions, expressing concerns or admitting uncertainty.

Effective communication within the surgical team involves more than just passing on information. It requires careful listening, clarification, mutual respect and a constant desire to improve interactions to ensure patient safety and well-being.

Managing disagreements and tensions in the operating theatre

The operating theatre is a high-tension environment where decisions are often taken quickly and the stakes are high. So it's not surprising that disagreements or tensions can arise between members of the surgical team. Here are a few strategies for effectively managing these situations while maintaining a professional and respectful atmosphere.

1. Stay calm:
    Emotional reactions can escalate an already tense situation. Take a deep breath, pause if you need to, and approach the situation calmly.
2. Listen Actively:
    Before responding or reacting, make sure you understand the other person's point of view. Listen without interrupting and avoid jumping to conclusions.
3. Clarify and Ask Questions:
    If you don't understand the other person's point of view or if any information is ambiguous, ask for clarification.
4. Avoid Direct Confrontation in Full Intervention:
    If a disagreement arises during a procedure, it may be preferable to stabilise the situation and postpone the discussion to a more appropriate time.
5. Use "I" rather than "You":
    Instead of saying "You didn't listen", say "I felt ignored". This avoids accusing the other person and opens the way to constructive dialogue.

6. Find Common Ground:
>   Even if you disagree, look for points on which you can agree. This creates a positive basis for discussion.
7. Call on a Neutral Mediator:
>   If tensions persist, it may be useful to call in a third party, such as a supervisor or mediator, to help resolve the conflict.
8. Think Before You Speak:
>   In the heat of the moment, it can be tempting to react impulsively. Take a moment to gather your thoughts before responding.
9. Encourage a Culture of Openness:
>   Create an environment where team members feel comfortable expressing their concerns or opinions without fear of reprisal.
10. Learn from Experience:
>   After resolving a conflict, take a moment to reflect on what happened. Are there lessons to be learned to avoid similar situations in the future?
11. Focus on training:
>   Encourage the team to take training courses on conflict management or interpersonal communication to reinforce the skills needed to manage tensions.
12. Be proactive:
>   If you identify potential sources of tension or disagreement, address them before they become a problem.

Managing disagreements and tensions in the operating theatre is essential to ensuring patient safety and team cohesion. By approaching each situation with empathy, open-mindedness and professionalism, it is possible to resolve conflicts and strengthen collaboration.

The importance of communication with the patient and family

The art of medicine goes beyond technical skills, and communication is one of its essential components. Effective communication with patients and their families can have a profound impact on the patient's experience, recovery and even clinical outcomes. Here's a look at why this communication is so crucial:

1. Building trust:
    Open and transparent communication establishes a relationship of trust between the healthcare professional and the patient, which is essential for a solid therapeutic partnership.
2. Anxiety reduction:
    Medical procedures, particularly surgery, can be stressful for patients. A clear and empathetic explanation can help reduce anxiety and worry.
3. Improving comprehension:
    Good communication ensures that patients and their families understand the nature of the condition, the treatment options and the associated risks and benefits.
4. Active participation in treatment:
    When patients are well informed, they can play an active role in their care, which can lead to better outcomes and greater satisfaction.
5. Expectation management:
    Communication helps to align the expectations of patients and their families with the realities and limitations of medical interventions.
6. Reducing medical errors:
    Exchanging relevant information with the patient can reveal crucial information, such as medical history or allergies, minimising the risk of errors.

7. Facilitating Informed Decision-Making:

    To give informed consent, patients need to understand all aspects of their treatment. Effective communication ensures that they have all the information they need to make informed decisions.

8. Emotional support:

    Acknowledging and validating the patient's emotions and concerns can provide vital emotional support, strengthening the therapeutic bond.

9. Care Transition:

    When the patient is transferred or discharged, clear communication with the family facilitates the transition of care and ensures continuity.

10. Conflict Resolution:

    If complications or problems arise, open and honest communication can help resolve tensions and avoid misunderstandings.

11. Cultural awareness:

    Taking into account the patient's beliefs, values and cultural concerns can help to personalise communication and improve the quality of care.

12. Promotion of Therapeutic Adherence:

    A well-informed patient is more likely to follow medical recommendations, which can improve long-term results.

Communication with patients and their families is at the heart of medical practice. It goes beyond the simple exchange of information to establish links, offer reassurance, guide choices and, ultimately, improve patients' quality of life. Adopting a patient-centred approach reinforces the importance of this communication in daily clinical practice.

Chapter 9:
RESOURCE MANAGEMENT
AND SAFETY IN ANAESTHESIA

Optimising use equipment and medicines

Efficiency and safety in the medical field rely heavily on the optimal use of equipment and medicines. Sound management can not only improve patient outcomes, but also reduce costs and minimise waste. Here's a seamless, integrated approach to optimising these crucial resources.

1. Training and Education:
   Providing ongoing training for healthcare professionals on the latest innovations and best practices in the use of equipment and medicines.
2. Protocols established:
   Develop clear protocols for the use of medicines and equipment, ensuring that procedures are consistent and based on the best available evidence.
3. Preventive maintenance:
   Carrying out regular checks and preventive maintenance on equipment to ensure that it is working properly and to extend its lifespan.
4. Stock management:
   Implementing an effective stock management system to monitor and manage the inventory of medicines and equipment, thus avoiding waste and shortages.
5. Regular assessment:
   Periodically review the effectiveness and suitability of the medicines and equipment used to ensure that they meet current and future needs.
6. Drug interactions:
   Use alert systems to monitor and prevent potentially dangerous drug interactions.

7. Recycling and Reuse:
   - Where safe and appropriate, consider recycling or sterilising and reusing equipment to maximise the use of resources.
8. Patient participation:
   - Educate patients on the appropriate use of medicines, stressing the importance of following prescriptions and avoiding self-medication.
9. Innovative technologies:
   - Adopting technologies such as automation and digitisation to improve the efficiency of medicines and equipment management.
10. Interdisciplinary collaboration:
    - Encouraging collaboration between the various medical teams to share knowledge and best practice in the use of medicines and equipment.
11. Incident Review:
    - Analysing and learning from incidents or errors relating to the use of equipment or medicines to continually improve practice.
12. Regulatory compliance:
    - Ensuring that all use of equipment and medicines complies with current regulations and guidelines to guarantee patient safety.

Optimising the use of equipment and medicines is an essential part of delivering high-quality healthcare. By focusing on training, proactive management and innovation, healthcare establishments can ensure that these valuable resources are used efficiently and safely.

Procedures and protocols to guarantee patient safety

Patient safety is the central pillar of healthcare. Ensuring safe care requires clear protocols, ongoing training and a safety-focused organisational culture. Here's an exploration of the procedures and protocols essential to keeping patient safety at the forefront.

1. Safety culture:
   - **Promoting an Open Culture**: Encouraging healthcare professionals to report incidents without fear of repercussions.
   - **Feedback**: Ensure a feedback loop after each incident to inform all staff of the lessons learned.
2. Patient identification:
   - Use several identifiers (name, date of birth, patient number) before any procedure or administration of medication.
3. Medication management:
   - **Secure storage**: Store medicines in locked or supervised areas.
   - **Double checking**: When administering critical medicines, use double checking by two professionals.
4. Infection prevention:
   - **Hand hygiene**: Implement strict hand-washing protocols.
   - **Isolation**: Isolate patients with transmissible infections to protect other patients and staff.
5. Training and Education:
   - Providing ongoing training on patient safety and the latest best practices.
6. Effective communication:
   - Set up protocols for transferring information when handing over from one team to another, to avoid forgetting crucial information.
7. Safe Surgery:
   - **Pre-Surgery Checklist**: Use checklists before, during and after surgery to ensure that all steps are followed.
   - **Marking of the surgical site**: Ensuring correct identification of the surgical site before the operation.

8. Technology and Equipment:
   Carrying out regular maintenance and quality checks to ensure that equipment is working properly.
9. Preventing falls:
   Assess patients' risk of falling on admission and implement appropriate interventions, such as the use of bed rails.
10. Informed Consent:
    Ensure that patients fully understand the procedures, associated risks and alternatives before any intervention.
11. Human Resources Management:
    Ensure adequate staffing levels and avoid work overload, which can contribute to errors.
12. Continuous Review and Improvement:
    Analyse incidents, carry out security audits and implement improvements based on lessons learned.

Ensuring patient safety requires a comprehensive and integrated approach that involves every member of the medical team. Errors may be inevitable, but with sound procedures and protocols, their frequency and impact can be reduced. Patient safety is a shared responsibility which, when prioritised, ensures better quality of care and greater patient confidence in the healthcare system.

Incident management and errors in anaesthesia

Anaesthesia is a medical field where the margins for error are narrow, with potentially serious consequences for patients. Managing incidents and errors effectively is crucial to minimising risk and learning from situations to avoid their recurrence. This section details the management of incidents and errors in anaesthesia.

1. Recognition and Immediate Response:
   Rapid response: When an error or incident is detected, the first priority is to intervene quickly to stabilise the patient.
   Immediate Notification: Immediately inform the surgical team and, if necessary, request assistance.
2. Documentation:
   Record in detail the circumstances of the incident or error, the measures taken in response, and the patient's condition after the procedure.
3. Transparent communication:
   With the patient and family: In compliance with ethical guidelines, inform the patient and family of the incident, the possible consequences and the corrective measures taken.
   Within the medical team: Discuss the incident with the team to learn immediate lessons and avoid repetition of the error in the near future.
4. In-depth evaluation:
   Root Cause Analysis (RCA): Undertake a systematic analysis to identify the underlying causes of the incident, rather than focusing solely on individual errors.
   Periodic assessments: Carrying out regular reviews of incidents and errors to detect trends or problem areas.
5. Training and Education:
   Use each incident as a learning opportunity for the whole team. Organise training sessions based on real-life scenarios to improve preparedness for similar situations.
6. Psychological support:
   Provide support to team members involved in the incident. Human error, while regrettable, is inevitable and support can help manage the associated guilt and stress.

7. Corrective measures:

Based on the findings of the PCA, implement systematic changes, whether this involves new training, changes to protocols or the purchase of new equipment.

8. Institutional transparency:

Maintain an error reporting system that protects the confidentiality of individuals while enabling the collection of data for continuous improvement.

Share lessons learned with other institutions or within wider medical networks to improve safety on a broader scale.

9. Review of Protocols:

Regularly review and adjust protocols and guidelines to ensure they are up to date with best practice and reflect lessons learned from previous incidents.

10. Commitment to Safety Culture:

Cultivate a culture where safety is a priority, where mistakes are treated as learning opportunities rather than as mistakes to be punished.

Incident and error management in anaesthesia is a multidimensional process that aims not only to rectify a given situation, but also to implement long-term changes to prevent recurrence. A proactive approach, combined with a strong safety culture, can greatly reduce risks to patients and increase confidence in the healthcare system.

Chapter 10:
INTERPROFESSIONAL COLLABORATION

Working with surgeons: understanding their needs and expectations

Successful surgery is the result of close collaboration between the surgeon and the nurse anaesthetist. Understanding surgeons' needs and expectations is crucial to ensuring patient safety and a smooth procedure. This section aims to shed light on the world of surgeons and suggest ways in which they can work together effectively.

1. The Dynamic Nature of Surgery:
    - **Understanding Surgical Techniques**: Recognising the different anaesthetic requirements depending on the complexity and duration of the surgery.
    - **Know the Key Points**: Be aware of crucial moments during the operation when the surgeon may require a change in anaesthesia.
2. Clear and effective communication:
    - **Before Surgery**: Discuss specific needs, concerns and expectations for the forthcoming operation.
    - **During Surgery**: Maintain open communication, reporting any changes in the patient's condition or anaesthetic parameters.
3. Mutual respect:
    - **Role Recognition**: Valuing each person's expertise while respecting the limits of their skills.
    - **Managing disagreements**: Handling disagreements professionally, always putting the patient's interests first.

4. Anticipating the Surgeon's Needs:
- **Material preparation**: Make sure that all the necessary equipment and medicines are ready and at hand.
- **Knowledge of habits**: Understanding surgeons' individual preferences and habits to facilitate cooperation.

5. Responsiveness to requests:
- Be prepared to adjust the anaesthetic to the changing needs of the surgery and to respond quickly to the surgeon's requests.

6. Combined Continuing Education:
- Participate in joint training sessions to understand the latest surgical and anaesthetic techniques and how they interact.

7. Post-op debriefings:
- After the operation, take a moment to discuss what went well and potential areas for improvement for future operations.

8. Understanding the Risks and Stresses Associated with Surgery:
- Recognise the pressure under which surgeons operate and offer support, whether clinical or emotional, where necessary.

9. Building mutual trust:
- Through open communication, mutual respect and close collaboration, develop a relationship of trust with surgeons.

Working closely with surgeons requires fluid communication, mutual understanding and respect for each other's skills and responsibilities. By focusing on patient safety and well-being, nurse anaesthetists and surgeons can overcome challenges and ensure optimal care.

Synergy with nurses
recovery room and intensive care unit

Once the surgery is over, the role of the nurse anaesthetist does not stop. Post-operative management, in particular the transition to the recovery room and eventually to intensive care, is a critical phase. Effective collaboration between the nurse anaesthetist and the nurses in these units is essential to ensure a safe and uncomplicated recovery for the patient.

1. The importance of communication:
    Passing on information: sharing all the relevant details about the anaesthetic, the procedures carried out and any complications encountered.
    Structured briefing: Use checklists or guides to ensure that all key points are covered during the briefing.
2. Understanding the Role of Recovery Room Nurses:
    Close monitoring: They are the first to detect signs of post-anaesthetic complications.
    Pain management: This involves managing postoperative pain and requires in-depth knowledge of the drugs administered during surgery.
3. Collaboration with the Intensive Care Unit:
    High-risk patients: For patients who require continuous monitoring after major surgery or because of co-morbidities, understanding intensive care protocols is crucial.
    Technical assistance: The nurse anaesthetist may be asked to assist with intubation or the placement of central access ports in these units.
4. Joint training:
    Participate in joint simulations and training to better understand the specific challenges faced by these nurses and to strengthen their skills in post-operative management.

5. Feedback:
   Establish a system where nurses can provide feedback on anaesthetic management, offering opportunities for continuous improvement.
6. Regular Coordination Meetings:
   Organise meetings to discuss protocols, share updates and address concerns or challenges.
7. Emotional and psychological support:
   Recognise the pressure under which these nurses work, particularly when faced with postoperative complications. Offer support and cooperation.
8. Continuity of care:
   Ensure that guidelines and recommendations are clearly communicated and followed, guaranteeing that the patient receives consistent and continuous care at every stage of their recovery.

The transition between the operating theatre, recovery room and intensive care unit is a complex journey for the patient. Effective synergy between the nurse anaesthetist and the nurses in these units ensures not only optimum safety but also an enhanced patient experience. The key is open communication, mutual respect and an understanding of each other's roles and responsibilities.

Working with pharmacists and other specialists

Anaesthesia is a complex, multifaceted medical practice that involves much more than the interaction between anaesthetist and patient. It often requires close collaboration with other specialists, including pharmacists, to ensure patient safety and effective care. This section explores the importance of this synergy and how collaboration can be optimised.

1. The Essentials of Pharmaceutical Collaboration:
   - **Drug selection**: Pharmacists provide essential expertise in drug selection, taking into account efficacy, drug interactions and possible allergies.
   - **Dosage and Administration**: They advise on appropriate dosages, routes of administration and timings, ensuring safe and effective anaesthesia.
   - **Stock management**: Ensuring the continuous availability of essential medicines through appropriate stock management in collaboration with the pharmacy.
2. Interaction with other specialists:
   - **Cardiologists**: In the case of patients with cardiac co-morbidities, a discussion with the cardiologist can guide the anaesthetic strategy.
   - **Respirologists**: For patients with respiratory pathologies, the advice of respirologists is crucial in avoiding postoperative complications.
   - **Nephrologists**: They play a key role for patients with kidney disease, advising on hydration, medication and post-operative management.
3. Multidisciplinary meetings:
   - These meetings bring together different specialists to discuss complex cases and draw up an optimal management strategy for the patient.
4. Cross-training:
   - Organise training sessions where the nurse anaesthetist can learn from the other specialists and vice versa, thereby strengthening mutual understanding and collaboration.
5. Protocols and Common Guidelines:
   - Develop joint guidelines with other specialties for patient management to ensure consistency and quality of care.

6. Availability for rapid consultations:
   Establish a direct communication channel for rapid consultations, enabling specialists to provide real-time advice during surgery.
7. Understanding Responsibilities:
   Each specialist brings unique expertise to the table. Recognising and respecting their skills and recommendations improves overall care.
8. Review of Complications and Outcomes:
   Hold review sessions where complicated cases or complications are discussed jointly, providing opportunities for learning and improvement.

Collaboration with pharmacists and other specialists is an often overlooked but crucial dimension of anaesthetic practice. It improves the quality of care, minimises risks and optimises patient outcomes. The key is open communication, mutual respect, an understanding of each other's skills and a willingness to work as a team for the benefit of the patient.

Chapter 11:
SPECIFIC PATHOLOGIES AND THEIR IMPLICATIONS FOR ANAESTHESIA

Managing patients with multiple co-morbidities

Anaesthetic management of patients with multiple co-morbidities is a delicate challenge. These patients are often more vulnerable to complications, and their management requires a multidimensional approach, meticulous anticipation and in-depth clinical expertise.

1. Preoperative assessment:
    Detailed Medical History: Gather full details of all existing conditions, medications taken and previous surgery.
    In-depth physical examination: A targeted examination to identify potential problems that could influence the choice of anaesthetic.
2. Multidisciplinary consultations:
    Working closely with other specialists to gain a full perspective and advice on the best approach for these patients.
3. Medical preparation:
    Optimisation: Adjust medications or treatments to stabilise comorbidities as far as possible before surgery.
    Specific tests: Depending on co-morbidities, additional investigations may be necessary, such as echocardiograms for cardiac patients.
4. Choice of anaesthesia:
    Opt for a method of anaesthesia that minimises risks while being effective for the planned surgery.

5. Intraoperative monitoring:
  - Advanced monitoring may be necessary for these patients to detect any complications or deviations from normal parameters at an early stage.
6. Medication management:
  - Pay attention to drug interactions, contraindications and potential side effects, taking into account co-morbidities.
7. Post-operative management:
  - **Close monitoring**: These patients may require prolonged observation in the recovery room or even admission to intensive care.
  - **Pain Management**: Ensuring that pain management is effective without aggravating their underlying conditions.
8. Preparing for the Exit:
  - Ensure a smooth transition to home care or an extended care unit with clear instructions on the management of co-morbidities and medication.
9. Communication:
  - Clearly inform patients and their families of the potential risks, benefits and management plan to ensure their informed consent.
10. Meticulous documentation:
  - Document all relevant details, decisions taken and the reasons behind them, for future reference and for other healthcare professionals involved.

Managing patients with multiple co-morbidities is one of the most demanding tasks in anaesthesia. It requires not only medical expertise, but also the ability to anticipate challenges, communicate effectively and make informed decisions to ensure patient safety and well-being at every stage of the surgical process.

Anaesthesia for patients suffering from rare diseases

Anaesthetic management of patients with rare diseases requires meticulous preparation, specialist knowledge and an approach tailored to each individual patient. These diseases, although uncommon, can pose unique anaesthetic challenges, increasing the risk of complications.

1. Understanding the Rare Disease:

   Research and documentation: finding out about the disease, its implications and the possible consequences for anaesthesia and surgery.

   Symptoms and Manifestations: Understand the symptoms and manifestations of the disease that can influence anaesthesia.

2. Preoperative assessment:

   Medical history: Gather details of the course of the disease, previous treatments and previous surgical procedures.

   Specialist Consultations: Working with GPs or specialists who manage the patient's illness to obtain specific information.

3. Preanaesthetic preparation:

   Specific drugs: Identify the drugs that should be avoided or preferred for these patients.

   Optimisation: Ensure that the disease is stabilised as far as possible before surgery.

4. Adapted anaesthetic techniques:

   Choice of Anaesthesia: Select an anaesthetic technique that is both safe for the specific disease and suitable for the surgical procedure.

   Advanced Monitoring: Some patients may require specialised monitoring due to their condition.

5. Intraoperative management:

    Increased vigilance: Be particularly vigilant for physiological changes that may not be typical of patients without this condition.

    Adaptability: Being prepared to adapt the anaesthetic technique according to the patient's response.

6. Post-operative management:

    Enhanced monitoring: These patients may require prolonged and careful post-operative monitoring.

    Communication with the medical team: informing the medical team of the specificities of the patient's illness and the anaesthetic management.

7. Patient and family education:

    Discuss the specific risks and precautions to be taken after surgery, taking into account the underlying disease.

8. Postoperative review:

    Organise follow-up meetings to assess the patient's response and identify areas for improvement for future interventions.

Anaesthetic management of patients with rare diseases requires not only clinical expertise, but also the ability to adapt and personalise the approach for each individual. The key is preparation, interdisciplinary collaboration and transparent communication to ensure patient safety and well-being.

Special considerations for elderly patients

With increasing life expectancy and medical advances, more and more elderly patients are undergoing surgery. Anaesthetic management of these patients presents specific challenges, as ageing is accompanied by physiological changes, co-morbidities and polypharmacy.

1. Age-related physiological changes:
   - **Cardiovascular**: Decreased cardiac reserve, increased vascular rigidity.
   - **Respiratory**: Decreased lung function, altered airway defence mechanisms.
   - **Renal**: Decreased renal function, altered drug metabolism.
   - **Neurological**: Increased sensitivity to anaesthetic agents, increased risk of postoperative confusion.
2. Preoperative assessment:
   - **Complete medical history**: Pay attention to comorbidities, medications and previous surgeries.
   - **Functional Assessment**: Evaluates the patient's ability to perform daily tasks, which can predict post-operative outcomes.
3. Medical preparation:
   - **Optimising Comorbidities**: Ensuring that existing conditions, such as hypertension or diabetes, are well managed.
   - **Medication**: Review the patient's medication to avoid interactions and reduce risks.
4. Choice of anaesthesia:
   - **Appropriate selection**: Opt for techniques that minimise the risks for the elderly patient, such as locoregional anaesthesia where appropriate.
5. Intraoperative management:
   - **Close monitoring**: Reinforced surveillance to detect any complications at an early stage.
   - **Prevention of Hypothermia**: Elderly patients are more susceptible to hypothermia in the operating theatre.
6. Post-operative management:
   - **Pain management**: Favour multimodal methods to minimise the side effects of opioids.

Confusion Monitoring: Elderly patients are more likely to develop postoperative confusion or delirium.

7. Early mobilisation:

Encourage early mobilisation to reduce the risk of complications such as pneumonia or deep vein thrombosis.

8. Effective communication:

Ensuring clear communication with patients and their families about the treatment plan, risks and benefits.

9. Care Transitions:

Coordinating the transition to post-operative care, whether at home or in a specialist unit, to ensure continuity of care.

The management of elderly patients requires particular sensitivity, thorough preparation and a global approach to optimise results and minimise complications. The aim is to ensure a safe and comfortable surgical experience for this vulnerable population.

Chapter 12:
EMERGENCIES AND EXCEPTIONAL SITUATIONS IN ANAESTHESIA

Anaesthesia in disaster and humanitarian crisis situations

Disasters and humanitarian crises, whether caused by natural disasters, armed conflict or epidemics, require a rapid and effective medical response. The provision of anaesthetic care in such situations is complex and presents many challenges.

1. Initial assessment:
    - **Needs Assessment**: What is the magnitude of the disaster? What types of injury or illness are prevalent?
    - **Available resources**: What equipment, medicines and staff are available on site?
2. Quick set-up:
    - **Setting up Emergency Operating Rooms**: Use tents, temporary structures or existing facilities.
    - **Sterilisation**: Sterilising instruments in often precarious conditions.
3. Resource limitations:
    - **Sub-optimal anaesthesia**: In some cases, we may have to make do with local anaesthetics or less ideal techniques.
    - **Pain management**: Opioids and other analgesics may be in short supply.
4. Staff training:
    - **Versatility**: In such situations, staff often have to take on several roles.
    - **Rapid training**: Train local staff or volunteers in the basic principles of anaesthesia.

5. Accrus risks:
   - **Infections**: Increased risk of infections due to surgery in non-sterile conditions.
   - **Complications**: Less monitoring and equipment means an increased risk of anaesthetic complications.
6. Interdisciplinary collaboration:
   - **Multidisciplinary teams**: working closely with surgeons, nurses, logisticians and other specialists.
7. Ethical and cultural aspects:
   - **Informed Consent**: Navigating situations where obtaining formal informed consent can be difficult.
   - **Respect for Cultural Norms**: Taking account of local beliefs and practices when providing care.
8. Psychological support:
   - **For Patients**: Recognising the trauma and stress experienced by patients and their families.
   - **For Staff**: Preventing burnout and providing psychological support for staff facing extremely difficult situations.
9. Transition to Long-Term Care:
   - **Rehabilitation**: Planning the transition of patients to post-operative and rehabilitation care.
   - **Ongoing training**: Ensure that local staff continue to be trained and equipped after the intervention teams have left.

Anaesthesia in disaster and humanitarian crisis situations requires flexibility, innovation and resilience. These interventions are crucial to saving lives in often chaotic and unfavourable contexts. The preparation, collaboration and dedication of staff are essential to providing quality care in these extreme situations.

Support an anaphylactic reaction

Anaphylaxis is a serious and potentially fatal allergic reaction. It can occur following the administration of many drugs and substances used during anaesthesia. It is therefore vital for nurse anaesthetists to be prepared to rapidly identify and manage such a situation.

1. Recognising symptoms:
    Cardiovascular: Hypotension, tachycardia or bradycardia, arrhythmia.
    Respiratory: Bronchospasm, cyanosis, hypoxia, laryngeal oedema.
    Cutaneous: Skin rash, urticaria, redness.
    Neurological: Malaise, confusion, loss of consciousness.
2. Immediate arrest of the guilty agent:
    If possible, immediately identify and stop the administration of the drug or substance suspected of causing the reaction.
3. Airway maintenance and ventilation:
    Intubation or Ventilation: Ensure adequate oxygenation and ventilation. Emergency intubation may be necessary in the event of laryngeal oedema.
    Supplemental Oxygen: Administer high concentrations of oxygen.
4. Cardiovascular stabilisation:
    Fluids: Intravenous fluids should be administered promptly to combat hypotension.
    Medication: Vasopressors such as adrenaline are often necessary.
5. Administration of adrenaline:
    Adrenaline is the drug of first choice for treating anaphylaxis. It must be administered immediately.
6. Antihistamines and corticosteroids:
    These drugs can be used to treat and prevent the progression of the anaphylactic reaction.

7. Management of Bronchospasm:
   Bronchodilators, such as salbutamol, may be administered to manage bronchospasm.
8. Continuous monitoring:
   Closely monitor vital signs, pulse oximetry, capnography and, if available, invasive blood pressure.
9. Cardiopulmonary resuscitation (CPR):
   In the event of cardiac arrest, start CPR immediately.
10. Post-Management:
   Once the situation has stabilised, it is crucial to transfer the patient to a unit where they can be monitored.
   Make sure that the patient, family and medical team are informed about the reaction and the potentially culprit drugs or substances.
   Further investigation to identify the culprit may be necessary.

Rapid and effective management of anaphylaxis by the nurse anaesthetist can mean the difference between life and death. Regular training and simulations in the management of these emergency situations are therefore essential.

Anaesthesia outside the operating theatre: emergency situations

Beyond the sterile walls of the operating theatre, the nurse anaesthetist may be called upon to intervene in emergency situations, whether in other areas of the hospital or even outside. These situations require not only technical skills but also the ability to adapt to less controlled environments.

1. Contexts where Anaesthesia Outside the Operating Theatre is Commonly Practised:

- **Imaging services**: interventional radiology, MRI, CT.
- **Endoscopy**: Gastroenterology, bronchoscopy.
- **Sterile rooms**: For immunocompromised patients.
- **Emergency**: Traumatology, resuscitation in the emergency room.
- **In the field**: disasters, war zones, rapid intervention.

2. Specific challenges:

- Non-sterilised environments: Increased risk of infection.
- **Limited equipment**: Absence of some of the block's usual features.
- **Reduced space**: Lack of mobility, difficulty accessing the patient.
- **Diverse medical team**: collaboration with professionals from other specialities.

3. Essential preparation:

- **Rapid Patient Assessment**: History, medication, allergies.
- **Equipment check**: Availability and operation of devices.
- **Communication**: Clear dialogue with the medical team and the patient.

4. Specific anaesthetic techniques:

- **Sedation**: Often used for short or painful procedures.
- **Local or Regional Anaesthesia**: Preferred for specific areas of the body.
- **General anaesthesia**: In more complex situations or for uncooperative patients.

5. Patient monitoring:

- **Monitoring**: Constant monitoring of vital signs.
- **Preventing complications**: Anticipating adverse reactions and respiratory problems.

6. Complication management:

- **Hypoxia**: Ensure adequate ventilation and oxygenation.

Allergic reactions: Prompt treatment with appropriate medication.

Cardiovascular complications: Managing arrhythmias, hypotension or hypertension.

7. Post anaesthesia:

Post-operation monitoring: Ensuring that the patient regains consciousness and is stabilised.

Transfer: Depending on the patient's condition, decide whether to admit him to an intensive care unit, recovery room or hospital.

Anaesthesia outside the operating theatre is a demanding practice that puts the nurse anaesthetist's versatility and adaptability to the test. Although it presents particular challenges, it is essential for ensuring quality care in diverse and often urgent situations. Continuing education and simulation are crucial in preparing these professionals for these unusual situations.

Chapter 13:
ANAESTHESIA AND SPECIAL POPULATIONS

Immunocompromised patients and transplants

In the vast world of medicine, the management of immunosuppressed and transplant patients poses unique challenges, especially when surgery requiring anaesthesia is required. The immunosuppressed state of these patients makes them particularly vulnerable to infections, drug reactions and other post-operative complications.

1. Understanding immunosuppression:
   Causes of immunodepression: Autoimmune diseases, chemotherapy, radiotherapy, immunosuppressive drugs, HIV, etc.
   Consequences for the immune system: Vulnerability to infection, delayed healing, altered inflammatory reactions.
2. Preoperative assessment:
   Medical history: reasons for immunosuppression, current treatments, history of infections, recent vaccinations.
   Clinical examination: Assessment of general condition, looking for active infections.
   Further investigations: Blood tests, chest X-ray, cultures if necessary.
3. Risks specific to anaesthesia:
   Drug reactions: Interactions with immunosuppressive drugs, increased risk of side effects.

- **Post-operative infections:** High risk due to the body's low defence capacity.
- **Healing**: Possible delayed healing of surgical wounds.

4. Anaesthetic preparation:
- **Antibiotic prophylaxis**: Administration of antibiotics before surgery to prevent infection.
- **Optimising nutritional status**: adequate nutrition to improve healing and immune response.
- **Mental Preparation of the Patient**: Reassurance, information on risks and benefits.

5. Intraoperative monitoring:
- **Intensive monitoring:** Close monitoring of vital signs, temperature and oxygen saturation.
- **Rigorous asepsis**: Maintaining a sterile environment to prevent infection.

6. Post-operative management:
- **Infection monitoring**: Monitoring for signs of infection, cultures if necessary.
- **Pain management**: Effective analgesia without further compromising the immune system.
- **Nutrition and hydration**: Ensure adequate nutrition to support recovery.

7. Transplant patients:
- **Knowledge of the graft**: type of transplant, date, possible complications.
- **Immunosuppressive drugs**: Dosage, drug interactions.
- **Risks of rejection**: Recognising the early signs of graft rejection.

Anaesthetic management of immunocompromised and transplant patients requires meticulous attention, rigorous preparation and increased monitoring. Every stage, from pre-operative assessment to post-operative recovery, must be adapted to minimise risks and ensure the best outcome for these particularly fragile patients.

Anaesthesia for patients with psychiatric disorders

Patients suffering from psychiatric disorders represent a specific population within the medical spectrum. Their particular needs, in addition to their medication and clinical history, require a nuanced and individualised approach when surgery under anaesthetic is required.

1. Understanding the Spectrum of Psychiatric Disorders:
   Overview of pathologies: Schizophrenia, bipolar disorder, major depression, anxiety disorders, PTSD, and others.
   Consequences for Perception and Cognition: Alterations in reality, vulnerability to anxiety or confusion.
2. Preoperative assessment:
   Psychiatric history: duration of illness, current and past treatments, episodes of hospitalisation, current symptoms.
   Medication history: Psychotropic medication, risk of drug interactions, compliance with treatment.
   Assessment of current mental state: stability, presence of acute symptoms, level of anxiety about surgery.
3. Risks specific to anaesthesia:
   Drug interactions: Potential interaction between anaesthetics and psychotropic drugs.
   Post-anaesthetic reactions: Increased risk of confusion, agitation and postoperative delirium.
   Pain Response: Altered perception of pain, amplified emotional response.
4. Anaesthetic preparation:
   Medication strategy: Adapt anaesthesia to minimise interactions and side effects.

- **Effective communication**: Ensuring that the patient understands the process and feels safe.
- **Psychological support**: Call in a mental health team if necessary to prepare the patient.

5. Intraoperative monitoring:
- **Monitoring for signs of agitation**: increased reactivity to stimuli, fluctuations in blood pressure or heart rate.
- **Adjusting anaesthesia**: Respond quickly to signs of stress or discomfort.

6. Post-operative management:
- **Delirium monitoring**: Recognise and treat signs of confusion or agitation quickly.
- **Pain management**: Adapting analgesic management to minimise emotional stress.
- **Post-operative communication**: Ensuring that the patient understands their situation and feels safe.

Anaesthetic management of patients with psychiatric disorders requires meticulous attention and interdisciplinary collaboration. Every phase, from preparation to recovery, must be approached with compassion, understanding and expertise to ensure the patient's safety and well-being throughout the surgical process.

Considerations for patients obese or bariatric

Anaesthesia for bariatric and obese patients presents unique challenges. These patients may have co-morbidities associated with obesity and anatomical and physiological changes due to surgery, requiring tailored anaesthetic management.

1. Obesity: Beyond BMI:
   - **Definition and Epidemiology**: Understanding the extent of obesity in the population.
   - **Associated co-morbidities**: Hypertension, diabetes, sleep apnea, heart disease, among others.
2. Preoperative assessment:
   - **Medical history**: Focus on pathologies associated with obesity.
   - **Surgical history**: Type of bariatric surgery, any complications, postoperative results.
   - **Respiratory function**: Risk of sleep apnea, reduced lung capacity, atelectasis.
3. Anatomical and physiological challenges:
   - **Airways:** Potential difficulty of intubation due to fat distribution.
   - **Cardiovascular system**: Increased cardiac workload, risk of arrhythmias.
   - **Drug metabolism**: Impaired distribution, metabolism and elimination of drugs.
4. Preparing for anaesthesia:
   - **Induction techniques**: Anticipate potential intubation difficulties.
   - **Patient positioning**: Ensure adequate ventilation and perfusion.
   - **Vascular access**: Ensure good cannulation, taking adiposity into account.
5. Intraoperative monitoring:
   - **Respiratory monitoring**: Risks of atelectasis and hypoxia.
   - **Haemodynamics**: Monitor cardiac overload and myocardial ischaemia.
6. Post-operative management:
   - **Respiratory management**: Risk of apnea, need for oxygen therapy.
   - **Pain management**: Assess the need for analgesics, taking into account drug metabolism.

Early mobilisation: Encouraging movement to prevent thromboembolic and respiratory complications.

The anaesthetic management of obese or bariatric patients requires careful planning, careful monitoring and close collaboration with the surgical team. A thorough understanding of the physiological changes and risks associated with obesity will help to ensure the patient's safety and well-being before, during and after surgery.

Chapter 14:
CHRONIC PAIN MANAGEMENT

Role of the nurse anaesthetist in pain clinics

Pain management is a fast-growing medical speciality. At the heart of this development, the nurse anaesthetist plays a major role by combining advanced clinical skills with a patient-centred approach to provide holistic care. Pain clinics are dedicated to the care of patients suffering from chronic, acute or post-operative pain, or pain caused by specific illnesses.

1. Understanding the Mechanisms of Pain:
    Types of pain: Distinguishing between nociceptive, neuropathic and psychogenic pain.
    Pain assessment: use of pain scales, pain history, triggers.
2. Intervention techniques:
    Nerve blocks: Peripheral and central blocks to relieve pain.
    Intrathecal therapies: Administration of drugs directly into the subarachnoid or epidural space.
    Radiofrequency and Neurolysis: Destruction of the nerves responsible for pain.
3. Administration of analgesic drugs:
    Opiates: Morphine, fentanyl and others.
    Non-opioid painkillers: Paracetamol, NSAIDs.
    Adjuvant medications: Antidepressants, anticonvulsants for neuropathic pain.
4. Holistic Approach to Pain Management:
    Complementary therapies: Acupuncture, massage, physiotherapy.

Psychological support: Identifying and treating the emotional component of pain.

5. Patient education:

Pain self-management techniques: relaxation techniques, meditation.

Knowledge of medicines: side-effects, risks of addiction, drug interactions.

6. Multidisciplinary collaboration:

Work with other health professionals: physiotherapists, psychologists, neurologists, etc. to provide comprehensive care.

Keeping up to date with the latest research: attending conferences, seminars and further training courses.

The nurse anaesthetist in a pain clinic is more than just a technician; they are an advocate, an educator, and often a pillar of support for patients desperately seeking relief. It is essential that the nurse anaesthetist possess not only strong clinical skills, but also an ability to empathise and understand in order to best serve this unique patient population.

Advanced techniques pain management

Pain, whether acute or chronic, can be extremely debilitating for patients. Advanced pain management is the culmination of decades of research, clinical practice and technological innovation. It aims not only to reduce pain, but also to improve patients' quality of life.

1. Interventional techniques:

Transcutaneous Electrical Neurostimulation (TENS): Use of electrical currents to modulate the perception of pain.

- **Spinal Cord Stimulation (SCS)**: Implantation of electrodes to block pain transmission.
- **Pulsed Radiofrequency:** Used to temporarily deactivate the nerves responsible for pain.

2. Advanced pharmacological approaches:
- **Analgesic Pumps:** Implantable pumps for administering analgesics directly into the epidural or intrathecal space.
- **Targeted treatments**: Use of specific drugs for specific types of pain, such as neuropathic pain.

3. Biological therapies:
- **Platelet Rich Plasma (PRP)**: Used to treat musculoskeletal pain thanks to the regenerative properties of the patient's own blood.
- **Cellular therapies**: Use of stem cells to promote healing and reduce pain.

4. Advanced Psychological Approaches:
- **Cognitive Behavioural Therapy (CBT)**: Helping patients understand and manage their reaction to pain.
- **Biofeedback**: Training patients to control certain physiological functions in order to manage pain.

5. Relaxation and meditation techniques:
- **Mindfulness meditation**: Focusing on the present moment to reduce the perception of pain.
- **Progressive Muscle Relaxation**: Gradually tense and relax muscle groups to relieve pain.

6. Complementary approaches:
- **Acupuncture**: The insertion of fine needles to stimulate specific points on the body.
- **Cold and heat therapy**: Using heat and cold to reduce inflammation and relieve pain.

Advanced pain management techniques require an in-depth understanding of pain mechanisms and specialist training. However, they offer new possibilities for treating patients suffering from refractory pain, and considerably improve their quality of life.

Working with other specialists in pain management

Pain management is a complex field that often requires a multidisciplinary approach to provide patients with comprehensive and effective care. Collaboration between nurse anaesthetists and other specialists is essential to develop and implement comprehensive treatment plans. This close collaboration provides a holistic vision that is tailored to each patient.

1. Rheumatologists:
   * *Assessment of musculoskeletal conditions*: Diagnosis and recommendations for pain of bone or joint origin.
   * *Collaboration in treatment*: Combining pharmacological and non-pharmacological therapies for optimal management.
2. Neurologists:
   * *Management of neuropathic pain*: Understanding nerve disorders and proposing appropriate treatments.
   * *Neurophysiological assessment*: In-depth tests to locate and quantify nerve damage.
3. Psychiatrists and psychologists:
   * *Psychological impact assessment*: Understanding how pain affects mood, sleep and general well-being.
   * *Therapeutic interventions*: Cognitive-behavioural therapies, biofeedback and other techniques to manage the psychological aspect of pain.
4. Physiotherapists:
   * *Physical therapy*: Exercises and manipulations to improve mobility and reduce pain.

Patient education: Advice on posture, movement and daily activities to prevent recurrent pain.

5. Clinical pharmacists:

Drug management: Advice on analgesic drugs, their interactions and side effects.

Adjuvant therapies: Suggestions for complementary agents to increase the efficacy of analgesic regimens.

6. Acupuncturists:

Traditional Chinese approach: Using acupuncture to reduce pain and stimulate healing.

Working together to combine care: Integrating acupuncture into an overall treatment plan.

7. Nutritionists:

Impact of nutrition on pain: Understanding how diet can influence inflammation and pain.

Dietary plans: Creation of specific diets to help reduce pain and promote healing.

By working closely with these specialists, the nurse anaesthetist can offer comprehensive, individualised care that goes beyond anaesthesia to ensure optimal pain management for each patient. This professional synergy enables a better understanding of the patient's needs, fluid communication and consistent implementation of treatment plans.

Chapter 15:
ENVIRONMENT
AND INFRASTRUCTURE
THE OPERATING ROOM

Optimal design and organisation of an anaesthetic room

A well-designed anaesthetic room is crucial not only for the efficiency of the process, but above all for patient safety. The layout, equipment and features of the environment must be meticulously thought through to ensure optimum care.

1. Spatial planning:
   - *Central zone*: Space for the patient, easily accessible from all angles.
   - *Circulation space*: Wide enough to allow easy movement of medical staff, without obstruction.
2. Lighting:
   - *Adjustable light*: Variable intensity to meet the needs of specific procedures.
   - *Emergency lighting*: In the event of a power cut, it must be instantly available.
3. Anaesthetic equipment:
   - *Anaesthesia machine*: Positioned for easy visibility and accessibility.
   - *Suction*: Functional, regularly tested and within easy reach.
   - *Monitors*: Ergonomic layout for quick reading of vital parameters.
4. Storage of medicines and consumables:
   - *Lockable cabinets*: For controlled drugs and potentially hazardous substances.

    Labelled drawers: organised according to frequency of use and product category.
5. Airway management:
    Dedicated storage: All sizes of laryngoscopes, masks, endotracheal tubes and other intubation devices must be readily available.
    Oral suction: Ready to use to remove secretions or obstructions.
6. Safety:
    Alarm systems: Functional and easily audible.
    Oxygen sensors: To prevent hypoxic situations.
    Fire extinguishers: Strategically placed to deal with potential fires.
7. Communications:
    Call systems: for rapid communication with other departments or specialists.
    Emergency telephones: For immediate access to emergency services.
8. Ergonomics and comfort:
    Ergonomic chairs: For staff, ensuring comfort during prolonged procedures.
    Controlled temperature: Maintains an appropriate ambient temperature for patients and staff.
9. Washing areas:
    Washbasins: With non-manual controls to reduce contamination.
    Disinfectant dispensers: Easily accessible for rapid hand hygiene.
10. Emergency equipment:
    Emergency trolleys: stored with resuscitation equipment, clearly labelled and regularly checked.
    Defibrillators: Charged and ready to use.

The design and organisation of an anaesthetic room reflect a commitment to safety, quality of care and efficiency. Every element, from the layout of furniture to the location of medicines, must be carefully planned to meet the needs of unforeseen situations and ensure optimum patient care at every stage.

Environmental safety and hygiene protocols

In the medical world, and particularly in the anaesthetic room, environmental safety and hygiene protocols are of the utmost importance. These play a vital role not only in preventing infections, but also in ensuring a safe and effective environment for patients and staff.

1. Infection control:
   - *Hand disinfection*: Encourage frequent hand washing and the use of alcohol-based disinfectants.
   - *Wearing protective clothing*: Systematic use of gowns, masks, gloves and goggles during procedures.
2. Equipment maintenance and cleaning:
   - *Disinfection protocols*: Regular cleaning of anaesthesia machines, monitors and other equipment with appropriate disinfectants.
   - *Regular maintenance*: Ensuring that equipment is working properly to prevent unexpected malfunctions.
3. Medical waste management:
   - *Waste separation*: Separate bins for biomedical waste, sharps and general waste.
   - *Safe disposal*: Follow local and national protocols for proper disposal.
4. Air quality and ventilation:
   - *HEPA filters*: Installation of ventilation systems with HEPA filters to eliminate fine particles and contaminants.
   - *Air quality monitoring*: Use of detectors to monitor oxygen levels and prevent leakage of gaseous anaesthetics.

5. Safety of floors and surfaces:
   - *Frequent cleaning*: Use disinfectant solutions to avoid cross-contamination.
   - *Anti-slip*: Keep floors dry to prevent falls.
6. Management of exposure to anaesthetics:
   - *Avoiding leaks*: Regular checks of connections and seals on anaesthesia machines.
   - *Adequate ventilation*: Avoid concentrations of gaseous anaesthetics in the air.
7. Safe storage of medicines:
   - *Lockable cabinets*: Keep medicines, particularly controlled medicines, in safe places accessible only to authorised personnel.
   - *Clear organisation*: Label and organise medicines to avoid medication errors.
8. Training and awareness-raising:
   - *Training sessions*: Organise regular training sessions for staff on health and safety protocols.
   - *Updates on best practice*: Ensuring that staff are aware of the latest health and safety recommendations.

Environmental safety and hygiene protocols are not just procedures, but a commitment to the well-being of patients and staff. In an environment as crucial as the anaesthetic room, every detail counts, and rigorous implementation of these protocols is essential to ensure the best possible care.

Resource management and supplies

The anaesthetic room is one of the pillars of a medical establishment. It is essential for many surgical procedures, both emergency and scheduled. Efficient management of resources and supplies is crucial, not only to guarantee patient safety, but also to ensure that operations run smoothly. From technical equipment to essential medicines, every element must be meticulously managed.

1. Drug inventory:
    Regular monitoring: Maintain an accurate inventory of available medicines and their expiry dates.
    Proactive ordering: Forecasting future needs based on planned surgeries and usual consumption.
2. Equipment maintenance:
    Maintenance schedule: Establish a regular maintenance schedule for each piece of equipment.
    Rapid repairs: A network of qualified technicians ready to intervene rapidly in the event of a malfunction.
3. Appropriate storage:
    Defined storage areas: Allocate specific areas for medicines, equipment and other supplies.
    Optimal conditions: Ensure that medicines and equipment are stored in ideal conditions to preserve their effectiveness.
4. Waste management:
    Safe disposal: Follow protocols for the correct disposal of medical waste.
    Waste reduction: Finding ways of optimising the use of resources to minimise waste.
5. Continuing education:
    Training on new equipment: Ensuring that staff are trained in the use of the latest equipment.
    Workshops on protocols: Organise sessions to inform staff of updates to protocols or the arrival of new drugs.
6. Working with suppliers:
    Strong partnerships: Establishing good relationships with reliable suppliers to ensure consistent supply.
    Strategic negotiations: Working on advantageous contracts, taking into account the establishment's long-term needs.

7. Emergency preparedness:
- *Emergency stocks*: Maintaining a reserve of medicines and equipment to deal with unforeseen situations.
- *Action plans*: Have clear protocols in place to respond quickly in the event of sudden shortages or other crises.

Managing anaesthetic room resources and supplies effectively is a delicate balance between anticipation and responsiveness. The unpredictable nature of medicine means that everything must be in place, at all times, to meet patients' needs. Rigorous management is therefore not only a question of logistics, but also a guarantee of confidence for patients and the entire medical team.

Chapter 16:
THE CHALLENGES OF TRAINING IN ANAESTHESIA

Development of training and certification programmes

The nurse anaesthetist profession is at the heart of patient care before, during and after surgery. It requires a high level of competence, clinical judgement and interpersonal skills. Over time, changes in medical techniques, technologies and patient needs have led training and certification programmes to adapt and modernise.

1. The birth of specialisation:
   The emergence of the role: How and why the role of nurse anaesthetist came about.
   The first programmes: The importance of formalising training to guarantee quality of care.
2. Technical and technological developments:
   Incorporation of technology: The integration of technological advances into the curriculum.
   Specialisations within anaesthesia: Training in specific techniques such as paediatric anaesthesia, cardiothoracic anaesthesia, etc.
3. Certification as a guarantee of quality:
   The importance of certification: Why is certification essential for nurse anaesthetists?
   Recent developments in certification criteria: how the bar has been continually raised to guarantee excellent quality of care.
4. Holistic approach to training:
   Beyond technique: The importance of communication, ethics and psychology in training.

Simulation as a teaching tool: How simulation has revolutionised training by providing hands-on experience without risk to patients.

5. Contemporary challenges and adaptations:

Specialisation vs versatility: How training programmes are adapting to the changing needs of the medical environment.

Continuous integration of recent research: Ensuring that training is always at the cutting edge of current knowledge.

6. International vision and exchanges:

Global comparisons: How do training programmes vary around the world?

Exchange and training opportunities abroad: The importance of diversity of experience in training.

7. The future of training and certification:

Adapting to technological advances: Anticipating the integration of new technologies, such as artificial intelligence, into the field.

Continuous updating of programmes: The importance of constant reassessment and adaptation to remain relevant and effective.

The evolution of training and certification programmes for nurse anaesthetists reflects the advances and challenges of the modern medical world. By remaining at the cutting edge of medical education, these programmes ensure that nurse anaesthetists are not only competent, but also leaders in their field, ready to offer the best possible care to their patients.

The importance of skills non-technical aspects of training

Anaesthesia, like many medical fields, is often viewed through the prism of technical skills, such as the ability to intubate a patient or administer medication correctly. However, to be truly effective in their role, nurse anaesthetists must also master a range of non-technical skills. These skills, which are often underestimated, are essential for ensuring patient safety, improving clinical outcomes and strengthening collaboration within medical teams.

1. Effective communication:
   - *The importance of listening*: How active listening can prevent medical errors and facilitate patient care.
   - *Communication with the team*: Working with surgeons, nurses and other professionals to ensure smooth care.
2. Decision-making under pressure:
   - *Clinical judgement*: The ability to quickly assess a situation and make informed decisions.
   - *Managing uncertainty*: how to navigate in situations where all the information is not available or is ambiguous.
3. Stress and fatigue management:
   - *Recognising your own limits*: The importance of knowing when to take a break or ask for help.
   - *Relaxation and resilience techniques*: Strategies for staying calm and focused, even in the most tense situations.
4. Teamwork and leadership:
   - *Creating a positive culture*: Promoting an environment where every member of the team feels valued and heard.
   - *Conflict resolution*: Techniques for resolving disagreements constructively.
5. Situational awareness:
   - *Problem anticipation*: The ability to foresee potential challenges before they arise.
   - *Maintaining a global vision*: Not getting lost in the details while keeping an overview of the situation.

6. Time and priority management:
  - *Organisation in a dynamic environment*: how to manage several tasks simultaneously without compromising the quality of care.
  - *Effective delegation*: Knowing when and how to delegate certain responsibilities.
7. Empathy and patient-centred care:
  - *Understanding the patient's needs and fears*: The importance of seeing the patient as a whole person, and not just as an illness or a procedure.
  - *Promoting dignity and respect*: Ensuring that every patient is treated with the respect and dignity they deserve.

Soft skills are a crucial part of nurse anaesthetist training. By combining these skills with solid technical training, nurse anaesthetists can provide comprehensive, empathetic and high-quality care, ensuring the safety and well-being of their patients.

Supervision, mentoring and knowledge transfer

1. Supervision: guaranteeing the quality of care
  - *The aims of supervision*: to ensure patient safety, reinforce the skills of novices and encourage ongoing clinical reflection.
  - *Supervision methods*: from direct observation to case review, how senior nurses effectively supervise junior nurses.
2. Mentoring: Inspiring and guiding the next generation
  - *The role of the mentor*: to be an adviser, a guide, a teacher and sometimes a confidant.
  - *The mentor-mentee relationship*: Building a relationship of trust, setting limits and defining clear objectives for professional growth.

3. Knowledge transfer: from theory to practice
  Teaching methods in anaesthesia: from simulation to real-life case studies, how to teach effectively in a dynamic clinical environment.
  The challenges of teaching: Overcoming barriers such as lack of time or generational differences to ensure effective transmission of knowledge.
4. Cultivating a continuous learning environment
  The culture of curiosity: Encouraging a lifelong learning attitude, where every experience, good or bad, is seen as an opportunity to learn.
  Constructive feedback: Learning to give and receive constructive criticism to encourage continuous improvement.
5. Evaluating and adapting training methods
  Measuring effectiveness: Use regular evaluations to ensure that knowledge transfer is effective and relevant.
  Innovating teaching: Exploring new methods and technologies to improve teaching in anaesthesia.

Supervision, mentoring and knowledge transfer are not just tools for training the next generation of nurse anaesthetists. They are also the means by which the profession renews, adapts and strengthens itself. By investing time and resources in these processes, nurse anaesthetists not only ensure quality care for today's patients, but also for those of tomorrow.

Chapter 17:
OUTPATIENT ANAESTHESIA

Principles and benefits outpatient anaesthesia

Ambulatory anaesthesia, also known as outpatient anaesthesia or day hospital anaesthesia, refers to surgical procedures in which the patient is admitted, operated on and discharged home on the same day as the surgery, without the need for an overnight stay in hospital. With advances in technology and improved anaesthetic methods, more and more operations are being carried out in this way. Let's take a closer look at the principles that guide this practice and its many advantages.

1. Principles of outpatient anaesthesia
   - *Appropriate patient selection*: Not all patients are suitable for ambulatory surgery. Inclusion and exclusion criteria are essential to ensure patient safety.
   - *Meticulous planning and coordination*: From preoperative preparation to discharge planning, everything must be meticulously organised.
   - *Specific anaesthetic techniques*: The use of short-acting anaesthetics, regional techniques and analgesics to minimise side effects and facilitate rapid recovery.
2. Benefits for patients
   - *Comfort and familiarity*: Patients can recover in the comfort of their own home, surrounded by their loved ones.
   - *Potentially faster recovery*: Familiar surroundings and the reduced stress of not having to be hospitalised can encourage a faster recovery.

114

Reduced risk of hospital-acquired infections: By avoiding an overnight stay in hospital, the risk of exposure to hospital-acquired infectious agents is minimised.

3. Economic benefits

Reduced costs: Less time spent in hospital means reduced costs for healthcare establishments and, potentially, for patients.

Increased throughput: Hospitals can treat more patients in outpatient surgery than in inpatient surgery.

4. Implications for the medical team

Changing dynamics: Rapid preparation, response and recovery require greater coordination and communication from the team.

Job satisfaction: Many find it rewarding to help patients recover quickly and go home the same day.

Ambulatory anaesthesia has revolutionised the way we think about surgery and anaesthesia. It represents a remarkable advance in the delivery of patient-centred care, while offering considerable economic benefits to the healthcare system. However, it is crucial to ensure that, while reaping the benefits of this approach, patient safety and well-being remain at the forefront.

Patient selection and preparation

The patient selection and pre-operative preparation processes are crucial stages in the surgical journey. These phases not only determine whether a patient is eligible for a procedure, but also lay the foundations for a safe and effective operation. Harmonisation of these stages is fundamental to optimising results and minimising risks.

1. Selection criteria: Who is the right candidate?

General state of health: The patient's medical history, chronic illnesses and current state of health must be assessed. Conditions such as heart, respiratory or kidney disease may influence the decision.

Nature of the surgery: Not all surgeries are suitable for all patients. Complexity, length of operation and anticipation of post-operative pain are all factors to consider.

Anaesthetic history: Previous reactions to anaesthesia, such as nausea or allergic reactions, should be noted.

Psychological assessment: The patient's ability to understand and follow post-operative instructions, as well as their level of comfort and anxiety about the operation.

2. Pre-operative preparation: making sure everything is in order

Medical consultations: Consultations with specialists may be necessary for patients with co-morbidities. For example, a cardiologist for a patient with a history of heart disease.

Laboratory tests: Blood tests, urine tests, X-rays or other investigations may be necessary to obtain a clear picture of the patient's condition.

Fasting: Patients are generally asked to fast for a certain number of hours before surgery to avoid complications during anaesthesia.

Medication: Some medicines should be stopped or adjusted before surgery, while others should be taken with a sip of water.

Patient education: Informing the patient about what to expect before, during and after surgery. This may include information on pain, mobility and post-operative care.

Careful patient selection and preparation are not mere formalities, but rather the first line of defence against complications and adverse outcomes. Open and transparent communication between the patient, the nurse anaesthetist and the surgical team is essential to ensure optimal care.

Post-operative management and follow-up

The post-operative phase is just as crucial as the pre-operative phase. While surgery is the central act, the post-operative period is when the patient really feels the impact of the operation. It is a delicate phase where the emphasis is on monitoring, pain management, preventing complications and promoting a rapid and complete recovery.

1. Initial post-operative monitoring
    - *Recovery room*: The first few hours after anaesthesia are vital. The patient's vital parameters are closely monitored, as is his or her ability to regain consciousness and breathe independently.
    - *Assessment of vital functions*: Continuous monitoring of blood pressure, heart rate, oxygen saturation and temperature to detect any abnormalities.
    - *Recovery from anaesthesia*: Assess the patient's mental clarity and ability to respond to stimuli.
2. Pain management
    - *Regular pain assessment*: Use of pain scales to quantify how the patient feels.
    - *Administration of analgesics*: Medication can range from paracetamol to opioids, depending on the intensity of the pain.
    - *Non-medicinal techniques*: Encouragement of early mobilisation, application of ice or use of relaxation techniques.

3. Preventing complications
- *Early mobilisation*: Helps prevent complications such as deep vein thrombosis or post-operative pneumonia.
- *Wound care*: Regular inspection of the surgical wound to detect any sign of infection or complication.
- *Hydration and nutrition*: Encourage patients to eat and drink as recommended to promote healing.
4. Patient and family education
- *Post-operative instructions*: Inform the patient about care at home, medicines to take, warning signs to watch out for and resumption of activities.
- *Follow-up appointments*: Schedule post-operative consultations to assess recovery and address any concerns the patient may have.
5. Transfer to specialised units or discharge
- *Discharge criteria*: Ensure that the patient is stable, can manage pain and understands all instructions before leaving hospital.
- *Rehabilitation and physiotherapy*: For some surgeries, rehabilitation is essential to regain mobility and function.

Post-operative management is not an isolated task, but an ongoing collaboration between the patient, the nurse anaesthetist and the entire medical team. Careful attention, clear communication and personalised care are the keys to a successful recovery.

Chapter 18:
PSYCHOLOGICAL ISSUES
IN ANAESTHESIA

Pre-operative anxiety :
understanding and reassuring the patient

The approach of surgery, even minor surgery, can be a source of worry, doubt and anxiety for many patients. The unknown, the fear of pain, the fear of complications, or even the simple idea of being put to sleep can be sources of anxiety. For a nurse anaesthetist, it is vital to understand this anxiety in order to offer adequate support and ensure the patient's well-being at every stage of the operation.

1. Recognising the signs of anxiety
   Physical symptoms: Trembling, sweating, palpitations, nausea or dizziness.
   Emotional symptoms: Irritability, crying, withdrawal, or expression of irrational fears.
   Behavioural symptoms: Repeated questioning, refusal to cooperate, or reluctance to follow instructions.
2. Common causes of pre-operative anxiety
   Fear of the unknown: Not knowing what to expect during and after surgery.
   Fears about anaesthesia: Fear of not waking up, of waking up during the operation or of possible complications.
   Concerns about the outcome: Fear of poor results, complications or a long convalescence.
   Personal concerns: worries about family, work or other responsibilities during the period of convalescence.

3. Strategies to reassure the patient
- *Open communication*: Encourage patients to express their concerns and answer all their questions clearly and honestly.
- *Pre-operative education*: Inform the patient about the operation, anaesthetic protocols and the recovery process. Familiarity can reduce fear of the unknown.
- *Relaxation interventions*: deep breathing techniques, visualisation, or even listening to soothing music.
- *Emotional support*: Providing a reassuring presence, allowing a relative to be present, or suggesting a consultation with a psychologist or counsellor.

4. Implications for medical staff
- *Ongoing training*: Ensure that all staff are trained to recognise and manage pre-operative anxiety.
- *Interdisciplinary collaboration*: Working with other members of the surgical team to ensure holistic management of patient anxiety.

Understanding and treating pre-operative anxiety not only benefits the patient's emotional well-being, but can also have positive implications for clinical outcomes. A calm and informed patient is more likely to co-operate, follow post-operative instructions, and may even experience a faster recovery. Empathy, patience and open communication are the keys to successfully navigating through these delicate moments.

Supporting patients after a traumatic experience

Witnessing or undergoing surgery that has not gone as planned, or dealing with unforeseen complications, can be traumatic for the patient. At such times, the nurse anaesthetist's ability to provide emotional and psychological support is essential to help the patient recover not only physically, but also emotionally.

1. Recognition and validation
   - *Active listening*: Providing a safe space for patients to share their feelings and concerns.
   - *Validation*: Acknowledge the patient's feelings without judgement. It is essential not to minimise their experience.
2. Clear and honest information
   - *Explain the situation*: Provide detailed information on what happened, why it happened and the steps taken to remedy it.
   - *Action plan*: Discuss the next steps for medical care and recovery.
3. Psychological support
   - *Referral to professionals*: Suggest a consultation with a psychologist or therapist specialising in trauma.
   - *Support groups*: Inform patients of the existence of support groups for those who have undergone traumatic medical experiences.
4. Regular monitoring
   - *Follow-up appointments*: Regular follow-up to assess the patient's physical and emotional recovery.
   - *Ongoing assessment*: Monitoring for signs of post-traumatic stress or other trauma-related disorders.
5. Self-care for the medical professional
   - *Supervision*: Seek opportunities for supervision or counselling to deal with personal feelings following traumatic medical incidents.
   - *Well-being practices*: Engaging in relaxation and stress-reduction activities to prevent burnout.
6. Prevention and learning
   - *Incident analysis*: Assess what went wrong and identify opportunities for improvement to prevent future incidents.

Ongoing training: Participating in training courses and workshops to improve clinical skills and communication techniques.

Supporting patients after a traumatic experience requires a holistic, patient-centred approach that takes into account not only their physical needs but also their emotional and psychological well-being. Open communication, empathetic listening and a willingness to provide the necessary resources are essential to help patients heal after such experiences.

The role of psychological support for anaesthetists

In the medical world, and particularly within anaesthetic teams, stress, pressure and high levels of responsibility are omnipresent. These professionals, who are on the front line when critical situations arise, are faced with a great deal of emotional pressure. Psychological support plays a vital role in ensuring their well-being and efficiency.

1. Recognising emotional weight
   - *Daily exposure*: Understand that nurse anaesthetists are exposed to life-and-death situations on a daily basis, and that they can be affected at any time.
   - *Impact on well-being*: Untreated emotions can lead to burnout, depression or other mental health problems.
2. Debriefing areas
   - *Post-operation debriefing*: offering regular opportunities for discussion and sharing after complex or stressful operations.
   - *Discussion group*: Creating a safe environment for colleagues to share and discuss their emotions.

3. Professional support
- *Psychological consultations*: professionals are available for individual consultations.
- *Specific training*: Organise training on stress management, resilience or communication in crisis situations.

4. Prevention strategies
- *Recognising warning signs*: Train staff to recognise the early signs of burnout or psychological distress in themselves and their colleagues.
- *Work-life balance*: Encouraging good time management and valuing breaks and holidays.

5. Building a culture of support
- *Open communication*: Valuing a culture where staff feel free to share their concerns without fear of judgement.
- *Recognition and appreciation*: celebrate successes and recognise the importance of everyone's work.

6. Research and development
- *Studies and publications*: Encourage studies into the mental health of anaesthetic professionals to better understand and anticipate their needs.
- *Integrating discoveries* : Applying new knowledge and techniques to improve well-being at work.

Ensuring the psychological wellbeing of anaesthetic staff is not simply a question of caring; it is a necessity to guarantee optimal patient care. A mentally healthy and supported team is an efficient and empathetic team, ready to face the challenges of everyday life.

Chapter 19:
COMPLEMENTARITY BETWEEN ANAESTHESIA AND INTENSIVE CARE

Basic principles of resuscitation

Resuscitation is the set of medical techniques designed to maintain or restore an individual's vital functions. The basic principles of resuscitation are essential for anyone working in the medical field, as they often deal with situations where every second counts.

1. Initial assessment
   - *Scene assessment*: Ensure that the environment is safe for the resuscitator and the patient.
   - ABCD of resuscitation:
     - Airway: Make sure the airway is clear.
     - Breathing: Check breathing and, if necessary, assist or replace this function.
     - Circulation: Check the pulse and, if necessary, initiate cardiac massage.
     - Defibrillation: Use a defibrillator if the patient is in cardiac arrest due to certain arrhythmias.
2. Advanced airway support
   - *Tracheal intubation*: Insert a tube into the trachea to secure the airway.
   - *Mechanical ventilation*: Using a device to assist or replace the patient's breathing.
3. Haemodynamic support
   - *Vascular access*: Establishing rapid access to the bloodstream to administer drugs or fluids.
   - *Vasoactive drugs*: Use medicines to support blood pressure and heart function.

4. Monitoring
- *Electrocardiography*: Monitoring the electrical activity of the heart.
- *Pulse oximetry*: Measures oxygen saturation in the blood.
- *Capnography*: Measuring exhaled CO_2 to assess ventilation.

5. Specific therapies
- *Thrombolysis*: Dissolving a clot blocking a blood vessel.
- *Therapeutic hypothermia*: Cooling the body to protect the brain after cardiac arrest.

6. Post-resuscitation
- *Stabilisation*: Ensure that the patient is stable after resuscitation.
- *Intensive care*: Transfer the patient to a specialised unit for close monitoring and ongoing treatment.

7. Ethics and decision-making
- *Patient consent and autonomy*: Respecting patients' wishes in terms of care.
- *Limiting and stopping treatment*: Recognising when it is in the patient's interest not to start or to stop an intervention.

Intensive care is a medical discipline that requires in-depth training, rapid decision-making and close coordination between team members. Although it is often associated with emergency situations, it is also part of an overall approach to care, support and respect for patient dignity.

Transferring the patient between the operating theatre and the intensive care unit

Transferring a patient from the operating theatre to the intensive care unit is a crucial stage that requires meticulous organisation, effective communication and multidisciplinary management to ensure the patient's safety and well-being. This is a time when the patient is particularly vulnerable due to recent surgical and anaesthetic interventions.

1. Pre-transfer preparation

Clinical assessment: Ensure that the patient is stable from a cardiorespiratory and haemodynamic point of view.

Communication: Informing the intensive care team of the patient's imminent arrival and the relevant details of surgery and anaesthesia.

Equipment preparation: Ensure that all vital support equipment (such as respirators) is working properly and ready for use.

2. The transfer process

Coordination: Determining who will be responsible for the patient during the transfer (usually the anaesthetic nurse or the anaesthetic doctor).

Safety: Make sure that the patient is firmly secured on the stretcher and that all tubes, catheters and wires are properly secured.

Monitoring: Continue to monitor the patient's vital functions during transfer.

3. On arrival in the intensive care unit

Transmission of information: Provide a detailed report to intensive care staff on the patient's current condition, details of the procedure, medication administered and any other relevant information.

Connecting to medical devices: Quickly connect the patient to the unit's equipment, such as the cardiac monitor, respirator, etc.

Initial assessment: The intensive care team must assess the patient immediately to ensure that he or she is stable and that any urgent needs are met.

4. Follow-up
  - *Documentation*: Document all details of the transfer, including times, people involved and any incidents or changes in the patient's condition.
  - *Continuous communication*: Maintain open communication between the operating theatre and the intensive care unit for any updates or changes concerning the patient's condition.

The immediate post-operative period can be one of the most critical for a patient. A well-organised and efficient transfer between the operating theatre and the intensive care unit is essential to ensure continuity of care and optimise patient outcomes. This requires close collaboration between anaesthetists, surgeons, nurses and the intensive care team.

Collaboration between nurse anaesthetists and intensive care physicians

Optimum medical care for patients, before, during and after surgery, is the result of close collaboration between a number of specialists. Among them, the nurse anaesthetist and the intensive care physician play key roles. Together, they work to ensure the patient's safety and comfort, while optimising their physiological state.

1. Complementary roles
  - *Pre-operative assessment*: The nurse anaesthetist is often involved in the initial assessment of the patient, taking a history and medication and identifying any problems. The resuscitator takes this assessment further, focusing in particular on the more complex aspects of the patient's co-morbidities.

Anaesthetic planning: While the nurse anaesthetist may propose an anaesthetic plan, the intensive care physician validates, adjusts and supervises its implementation, taking into account the implications for the post-operative period.

2. Teamwork in the operating theatre

Induction and maintenance of anaesthesia: The nurse anaesthetist is often responsible for administering anaesthetic drugs and monitoring vital signs, under the supervision and guidance of the resuscitating doctor.

Complication management: In the event of a complication, the anaesthetic nurse and the intensive care doctor work together to stabilise the patient quickly.

3. Post-operative period

Transfer to the intensive care unit (ICU): This phase is crucial and often involves both the anaesthetist nurse, who monitored the patient in the operating theatre, and the resuscitation doctor, who will take charge of the patient in the ICU.

Follow-up in the ICU: While the nurse anaesthetist may provide initial follow-up, the resuscitation doctor will take over post-operative management, looking after the patient's pain, breathing and general recovery.

4. Communication and training

Regular exchanges: Regular meetings between the two professionals enable complex cases to be discussed, protocols to be fine-tuned and optimum collaboration to be ensured.

Continuing training: Joint training courses are beneficial for strengthening synergy, sharing knowledge and staying at the cutting edge of medical advances.

Collaboration between the nurse anaesthetist and the resuscitation doctor is fundamental to ensuring that operations run smoothly and patients are safe. This partnership must be based on respect, trust and communication to ensure holistic and effective patient care.

Chapter 20:
DRUGS IN ANAESTHESIA: NEWS AND PERSPECTIVES

New anaesthetic agents on the market

Anaesthesia is a constantly evolving medical speciality, and pharmaceutical research is continually aimed at developing anaesthetic agents that are safer, more effective and better tolerated by patients. Here is an overview of recent developments and emerging agents in the field of anaesthesia. Note that this overview is based on my knowledge up to January 2022, and it is crucial to consult current resources for up-to-date information.

1. Anaesthetic inhalers
New inhalers are being developed to offer faster recovery, fewer side effects and a smaller environmental footprint.

    Desflurane, Sevoflurane, Isoflurane: Although these agents are not new in themselves, advances are being made to improve their administration and minimise their impact on the environment.

2. Intravenous agents

    Remimazolam: An ultra-rapid-acting benzodiazepine with the advantage of a short half-life and rapid elimination, which could lead to a quicker awakening.

    Dexmedetomidine: A sedative that acts on alpha-2 adrenergic receptors, providing sedation without respiratory depression.

3. Local nerve blocks

    New liposomes: Research is aimed at developing liposomal preparations of drugs such as bupivacaine, enabling prolonged release and therefore longer-lasting analgesia without the need for continuous infusions.

4. Non-opioid agents for pain management
    Tapentadol: Acting as both an opioid agonist and a norepinephrine reuptake inhibitor, it offers an option for both acute and chronic pain.
    Agents targeting NMDA receptors: Agents such as ketafol (a combination of ketamine and propofol) are being studied for their analgesic potential.
5. Environmental considerations
Research is also focusing on reducing the carbon footprint of anaesthetic agents, in particular by optimising delivery systems to minimise greenhouse gas emissions.

It is crucial for all nurse anaesthetists and anaesthetist-resuscitators to keep abreast of the latest developments, not only to provide the best possible care, but also to anticipate changes in day-to-day practice. Attending conferences, reading specialist journals and getting involved in professional associations are all ways of staying at the cutting edge of the speciality.

Trends in sedation and nerve blocks

Anaesthetic practice is constantly evolving, and new trends in sedation and nerve blocks have emerged in recent years. These trends have been influenced by technological advances, clinical research and a better understanding of patients' needs.

1. Sedation :
    Minimal sedation: Conscious sedation, where the patient remains awake but relaxed, has become popular for many procedures, enabling a faster recovery with fewer side effects.
    Non-opioid sedation agents: Research is aimed at reducing dependence on opioids for sedation. Agents

such as propofol, dexmedetomidine and remimazolam offer interesting options.

- **Oral sedation:** For shorter or less invasive procedures, oral sedative agents are increasingly used, reducing the need for intravenous administration.

2. Nerve blocks :

- **Ultrasound guidance:** The use of ultrasound to guide nerve block injections has revolutionised this practice. It increases the accuracy of anaesthetic placement, reduces the risk of complications and improves the efficiency of the block.
- **Continuous nerve block catheters:** These catheters provide continuous analgesia after painful surgery, offering better pain management without the need for prolonged use of opioids.
- **Peripheral nerve blocks vs central blocks:** Peripheral nerve blocks, such as brachial plexus blocks or fascial blocks, are increasingly preferred for specific surgical procedures, reducing the need for more invasive central techniques such as spinal anaesthesia.
- **New adjuvants:** Agents such as dexmedetomidine and dexamethasone are added to local anaesthetics to prolong the duration of nerve block analgesia.

The evolution of sedation and nerve block techniques reflects the general trend towards more individualised, patient-centred medicine. With advances in technology and the adoption of new methods, nurse anaesthetists and resuscitation anaesthetists can offer quality care, while ensuring the safety and comfort of their patients.

Resistance-related issues to medicines and alternatives

Advances in anaesthesia, as in other medical fields, are coming up against the emergence of drug resistance. This resistance represents a major challenge for healthcare professionals and can have direct implications for the effectiveness of surgical procedures and patient safety.

1. Understanding drug resistance :
    Resistance mechanisms: Over time, certain bacteria and other micro-organisms develop mechanisms to counter the effects of drugs. This is often the result of excessive or inappropriate use of drugs.
    Consequences for anaesthesia: Drug resistance can affect the ability of anaesthetics to produce the desired effect, which may necessitate the use of higher doses or alternative drugs, with potentially increased risks for the patient.

2. Specific issues in anaesthesia :
    Antibiotic resistance: Prophylactic antibiotics are commonly used in surgical procedures to prevent infection. Antibiotic resistance can compromise this strategy, increasing the risk of post-operative infections.
    Resistance to anaesthetic agents: Although less common, some patient populations may have an increased tolerance to certain anaesthetic agents, requiring adjustments to anaesthetic protocols.

3. Alternatives and strategies in the face of resistance :
    Research into new drugs: It is essential to develop new anaesthetic and analgesic drugs to deal with resistance.
    Optimising protocols: Judicious use of existing drugs, by combining agents or modifying dosages,

can help maximise their efficacy while minimising the development of resistance.

Monitoring and education: Monitoring resistance trends and educating healthcare professionals on the appropriate use of drugs is crucial.

Non-drug therapies: Adopting alternative techniques, such as nerve blocks, non-opioid sedation or relaxation techniques, can reduce dependence on certain drugs and minimise the risk of resistance.

The emergence of drug resistance represents a significant challenge for the field of anaesthesia. However, through interdisciplinary collaboration, ongoing research and judicious use of available resources, healthcare professionals can continue to provide safe and effective care to their patients.

Chapter 21:
QUALITY AND CONTINUOUS IMPROVEMENT IN ANAESTHESIA

Management principles quality in healthcare

Quality management in healthcare aims to ensure that healthcare is safe, effective, patient-centred, timely, efficient and equitable. It is based on a systemic approach geared towards continuous improvement, with the emphasis on preventing errors rather than correcting them. Here is an overview of the fundamental principles that guide this approach:

1. Focus on the patient :
   Understanding patients' needs and expectations: Care must be designed around the patient, taking into account their preferences, needs and values.
   Promoting patient participation: Involving patients in decision-making about their care, and encouraging a partnership between patients, their families and healthcare professionals.

2. Evidence-based approach :
   Use of the best available evidence: Adopt clinical practices based on current and relevant scientific evidence to ensure the effectiveness of interventions.
   Innovation and research: Encouraging clinical research and innovation to constantly improve the quality of care.

3. Continuous improvement :

Evaluation and feedback: Use measurement and evaluation tools to identify areas for improvement.

Implement corrective actions: Once the problems have been identified, implement actions to resolve them and prevent their recurrence.

4. Committed leadership :

Promoting a culture of quality: Managers must commit to promoting an organisational culture that values the quality and safety of care.

Training and education: Ensure that all staff are properly trained in the principles of quality and safe care.

5. Transparent communication :

Sharing information: Facilitating communication between all the players in the healthcare system to ensure coordinated and effective patient care.

Reporting incidents: Encourage the reporting of incidents and errors to learn from them and improve systems.

6. Teamwork and collaboration :

Promoting interdisciplinary work: Encouraging collaboration between different healthcare professionals to provide comprehensive patient care.

Partnerships: Working with other institutions and organisations to share best practice and resources.

7. Fairness :

Guaranteeing access: Ensuring that all patients, whatever their origin or situation, have access to quality care.

Personalising care: Tailoring care to the specific needs of each patient, while guaranteeing equal treatment for all.

Quality management in healthcare requires an ongoing commitment from healthcare professionals, managers and patients themselves. It aims not only to improve clinical care, but also to ensure a positive patient experience throughout the care journey.

Assessment methodologies and improving performance

In the medical environment, and for nurse anaesthetists in particular, performance evaluation and improvement are crucial to guaranteeing the safety and quality of care. Various methodologies are used to achieve this objective. Let's find out more about these methods:

1. Clinical audit :
   Definition and objectives: A clinical audit is a systematic review of the provision of care, compared against clear criteria. Its aim is to improve the quality of patient care.
   Procedure: Identify an audit question or topic, define criteria and standards, collect and analyse data, then implement changes.

2. Mortality and morbidity review (MMR) :
   Objective: To systematically examine deaths and complications occurring in a department or institution.
   Procedure: Analyse the cases, determine whether improvements can be made and implement corrective actions if necessary.

3. PDCA cycle (Plan, Do, Check, Act) :
   Plan: Identify a problem or an opportunity for improvement, then draw up an action plan.
   Do: Implement the plan on a small scale to test it.

Check: Evaluate results and compare performance before and after.

Take action: Based on the results, decide whether to implement the plan on a large scale or revise it.

4. Six Sigma :

Objective: A structured approach to improving performance by eliminating errors and defects.

Procedure: Uses statistical tools to identify processes requiring improvement, then optimises them.

5. Key performance indicators (KPI) :

Definition: Specific indicators that help an organisation measure its performance against its strategic objectives.

Use: KPIs are used to assess current performance, define future targets and implement corrective actions.

6. Peer reviews :

Objective: To provide feedback on individual performance based on observations of colleagues.

Procedure: Professionals assess their peers on the basis of pre-established criteria. This method may be formal or informal.

7. Benchmarks or benchmarking :

Definition: Comparing the performance of an organisation or unit with that of recognised best practice or standards.

Use: Identify performance gaps and implement strategies to meet or exceed these standards.

8. Patient satisfaction assessments :

Objective: To measure patient satisfaction in order to assess the quality of care.

Procedure: Use of questionnaires, interviews or other methods to gather patients' opinions.

Each of these methodologies offers a unique perspective on performance. By combining them and adapting them to the specific needs of an institution or department, it is possible to obtain a complete picture of performance and identify areas for improvement. The key is to engage in a continuous improvement process, always ensuring that the patient is at the centre of attention.

Feedback and incident analysis

In the medical field, and particularly in anaesthesia, even minor incidents can have serious consequences for patients. Feedback and analysis of incidents are therefore essential to improving the quality and safety of care. Let's take a fluid, in-depth look at these elements.

1. The importance of feedback :
Feedback is not just about mistakes or failures. It's a learning process that allows us to evaluate concrete situations, learn from them and improve future practices. In the world of anaesthesia, feedback is crucial to avoid repeating the same mistakes.

2. A culture of safety, not guilt :
To encourage the sharing of incidents or mistakes, it is essential to establish a culture where safety is a priority and where professionals feel free to share their experiences without fear of negative repercussions. It is by acknowledging and understanding our mistakes that we can truly move forward.

3. Incident analysis methodology :

Gathering information: Immediately after an incident, it is essential to document all relevant details, including the events leading up to the incident, the people involved, the equipment used, etc.

Causal analysis: Rather than simply identifying what went wrong, it is crucial to understand why. Root cause analysis can help identify systemic or organisational issues that contributed to the incident.

Development of solutions: Based on the analysis, recommendations are made to prevent similar incidents from occurring in the future.

4. Sharing lessons :
Once the analysis has been completed, it is essential to share the conclusions and lessons learned with the team, and even with the whole institution. This can take the form of team meetings, training courses or publications.

5. Continuous improvement :
The loop does not stop once the incident has been analysed. Recommendations must be implemented, monitored and evaluated to ensure that they are effective.

6. Technological aids :
Technological tools, such as electronic reporting systems, can facilitate the collection, analysis and monitoring of incidents. These systems can also help to identify trends or recurring problems.

7. Patient involvement :
Patients, or their families, can provide valuable perspectives on incidents. By involving them in the analysis process, we can obtain a more complete view of the event and build confidence.

Every incident, however regrettable, offers a unique opportunity to learn and improve. By adopting a systematic and caring approach to incident analysis, nurse anaesthetists and their teams can continually improve the safety and quality of the care they provide.

Chapter 22:
HISTORICAL PERSPECTIVES
OF ANAESTHESIA

The evolution of anaesthesia
through the ages

Since the earliest days of civilisation, mankind has sought ways to relieve pain, particularly during medical or surgical procedures. Anaesthesia, as we know it today, is the result of millennia of experimentation, chance discoveries and medical innovations. Let's travel through time to trace the evolution of this essential medical discipline.

1. Ancient origins :
Before the advent of modern anaesthesia, ancient civilisations used primitive methods to alleviate pain. The Egyptians, for example, used opiates and alcohols to induce a state of unconsciousness. The Chinese, meanwhile, were perhaps the first to practise acupuncture for analgesic purposes.

2. The Middle Ages and the Renaissance :
During these periods, medicine took tentative steps. Mixtures of herbs, alcohols and opiates were commonly used to relieve pain, although their effectiveness varied. Attempts, often disastrous, to use substances such as mandrake or belladonna were common.

3. The 19th century: The age of innovation :
   Ether and chloroform: In 1846, the first successful surgical procedure using ether was performed in Boston. Shortly afterwards, chloroform was introduced as an alternative. These substances have

revolutionised surgery, although they have their own risks and drawbacks.

Cocaine: Discovered as a local anaesthetic in ophthalmology, it paved the way for other, safer local anaesthetics.

4. The 20th century: Towards safer anaesthesia :

Introduction of barbiturates: In the 1930s, these drugs were introduced for anaesthetic induction, offering more control than inhaled agents.

Development of regional anaesthesia: With the introduction of drugs such as lidocaine, techniques such as spinal anaesthesia and epidural anaesthesia became popular.

Monitoring equipment: The second half of the century saw the development of sophisticated devices to monitor the patient's condition, thereby increasing safety.

5. The 21st century: personalisation and precision :

With the advent of genomics and personalised medicine, anaesthesia has become even more targeted. Rapid-acting anaesthetic agents, ultrasound-guided regional anaesthesia techniques, and a better understanding of drug interactions and side effects have all contributed to making anaesthesia safer and more effective than ever before.

The history of anaesthesia is littered with trial and error, discovery and innovation. From primitive and often dangerous practices to a sophisticated and safe medical discipline, anaesthesia has come a long way, bearing witness to mankind's ceaseless quest for pain relief and patient safety.

Pioneers and landmark discoveries

The practice of anaesthesia has been shaped by a series of discoveries and innovations that have revolutionised medicine and surgery. Behind each breakthrough there have been visionary individuals who have dared to push back the boundaries of what is possible. Let's take a look at some of these pioneers and their landmark contributions.

1. Horace Wells (1815-1848):
   Contribution: The use of nitrous oxide (or laughing gas) as an anaesthetic agent.
   Wells, a dentist, was the first to use nitrous oxide to extract a tooth painlessly. Although his first public demonstrations were fraught with controversy, his discovery laid the foundations of modern anaesthesia.

2. William Thomas Green Morton (1819-1868):
   Contribution: The first successful use of ether as an anaesthetic.
   Morton successfully demonstrated the use of ether for anaesthesia in 1846 at the Massachusetts General Hospital. This demonstration, now famous as "Ether Day", marked a turning point in surgery.

3. James Young Simpson (1811-1870) :
   Contribution: The introduction of chloroform in anaesthesia.
   Simpson, a Scottish obstetrician, was the first to recognise the anaesthetic properties of chloroform and to use it to relieve the pain of childbirth.

4. Carl Koller (1857-1944) :
   Contribution: The discovery of the anaesthetic properties of cocaine for eye surgery.

Koller, an ophthalmologist, introduced cocaine as a local anaesthetic in ophthalmology, revolutionising eye surgical procedures.

5. John Snow (1813-1858):

Contribution: A pioneer in the controlled administration of anaesthetics.

Also known for his work in epidemiology, Snow improved the methods of administering chloroform and ether, and in particular administered chloroform to Queen Victoria during childbirth.

6. Virginia Apgar (1909-1974) :

Contribution: Development of the "Apgar Score".

Apgar, an anaesthetist and paediatrician, developed the Apgar score to quickly assess the health of newborn babies, a procedure still used today in delivery rooms around the world.

7. Sir Ivan Magill (1888-1986):

Contribution: Innovation in thoracic anaesthesia.

Magill developed a series of instruments and techniques for tracheal intubation, including the famous Magill forceps, which are still in use today.

These pioneers, among others, laid the foundations of modern anaesthesia. Their curiosity, perseverance and ingenuity improved the safety and effectiveness of medical procedures, benefiting millions of patients around the world.

Lessons learned and influence on current practice

The history of anaesthesia is littered with resounding successes, dismal failures, bold experiments and progressive developments. By examining this rich history, it is possible to discern essential lessons that continue to shape current practice. These lessons transcend time and technology, reminding professionals of the fundamental principles of their profession.

1. Safety first:
Tragic failures, such as deaths due to overdose or administration errors, have reinforced the need for careful patient assessment and monitoring during anaesthesia. Current practices, with their strict protocols and advanced monitoring equipment, reflect this lesson.

2. The need for continuing education :
As new agents and techniques were discovered, it became clear that initial training was insufficient. Today, continuing education, regular certification and simulations have become the norm, ensuring that anaesthetists are always at the cutting edge of their profession.

3. The importance of interprofessional collaboration
Figures such as John Snow, who worked closely with surgeons, have shown that anaesthesia does not take place in a vacuum. Today, teamwork between anaesthetists, surgeons, nurses and other healthcare professionals is essential to ensure optimal patient care.

4. Adaptability in the face of the unknown :
Faced with new or unexpected situations, anaesthetists in the past have often had to improvise. This ability to adapt remains crucial today, particularly in emergency situations or with patients presenting complex medical challenges.

5. Ethics and informed consent :
Early anaesthesia was sometimes administered without the patient's full consent. The resulting scandals and consequences have highlighted the crucial importance of

informed consent, a practice now deeply embedded in medical procedures.

6. Responsible innovation and experimentation :
While boldness and innovation have been essential to progress in anaesthesia, they must be balanced by an ethical and responsible approach. Modern clinical research in anaesthesia is therefore rigorously regulated, ensuring that new methods are both safe and effective.

7. The importance of communication and education :
The pioneers of anaesthesia were also ardent advocates of their profession, educating the public and other healthcare professionals about the benefits and risks of anaesthesia. Today, communication with patients, their families and the medical team remains a cornerstone of anaesthetic practice.

These lessons from the past are not simply historical accounts; they form the foundation on which modern anaesthetic practice rests. They remind today's professionals of the seriousness of their responsibility and guide them in their ongoing quest for excellence.

Chapter 23:
CAREER DEVELOPMENT

Academic career
and continuing education

Anaesthesia, as a medical speciality, requires a high level of skill, precision and knowledge. Academic background and continuing education play a crucial role in ensuring that professionals in this field are well equipped to provide safe and effective care. Here is an overview of the typical academic pathway and the importance of continuing education in this specialty.

1. Initial training :
   - **Pre-medical studies**: As with other medical professions, a candidate in anaesthesia often starts with a university pre-medical training covering the basics of the biological, chemical and physical sciences.
   - **Medical school**: After obtaining a pre-medical diploma, students enter medical school for a four- to six-year course (depending on the country), where they obtain their medical diploma.

2. Specialised training :
   - **Internship**: After medical school, aspiring anaesthetists generally enter an internship programme lasting one to two years, focusing on general clinical practice.
   - **Anaesthesia residency**: Depending on the internship, an anaesthesia residency is required. This generally lasts between three and five years and

focuses exclusively on anaesthesia and its sub-specialities.

3. Certification and approval :
- **Certification exam**: After residency, anaesthetists often have to pass an exam to become certified in their specialty.
- **Accreditation**: Depending on the jurisdiction, an anaesthetist may also need accreditation or a licence to practise.

4. Continuing education :
Medicine, and anaesthesia in particular, is a constantly evolving field. New techniques, drugs and technologies emerge regularly. To keep up to date:
- **Courses and workshops**: Workshops, seminars and courses are regularly organised by professional associations or academic institutions.
- **Clinical simulations**: With the advent of simulation technology, anaesthetists can practice complex scenarios in a safe environment.
- **Re-certification**: Some countries or regions require anaesthetists to be re-certified every few years, which may involve passing exams or proving a certain amount of continuing education.
- **Reading and research**: Regular reading of professional journals and participation in research projects may also be encouraged or required.

5. Sub-specialities :
As with other medical fields, anaesthesia has several sub-specialties, such as paediatric anaesthesia, cardiac anaesthesia or pain medicine. Each of these sub-specialties may require additional training and certification.

An anaesthetist's academic and professional career is long and demanding. However, this rigour ensures that patients receive the best possible care when they are at their most vulnerable. Continuing education is not only an ethical imperative, it is essential to ensure the safety, efficacy and evolution of anaesthetic practice.

Specialisation opportunities in the field of anaesthesia

Anaesthesia is a vast medical field that offers many opportunities for specialisation. Each of these specialities requires specific training and expertise to meet the particular needs of patients. Here is an overview of the main sub-specialities in anaesthesia:

1. Paediatric anaesthesia :
   This speciality focuses on the anaesthetic management of neonates, infants, children and adolescents.
   It requires in-depth knowledge of the physiology and diseases specific to this age group.

2. Cardiac anaesthesia :
   Focuses on patients undergoing cardiac surgery, including bypass surgery and valve operations.
   Cardiac anaesthetists are trained to manage complex haemodynamic situations and often use transoesophageal echocardiography.

3. Obstetric anaesthesia :
   Focused on caring for women during labour and birth.
   Includes management of epidurals, spinal anaesthesia and other forms of anaesthesia for caesarean sections.

4. Pain medicine :
   Focuses on the management and treatment of chronic pain.

Procedures often include nerve blocks, epidural injections and the implantation of drug pumps.

5. Neurosurgical anaesthesia :
   - For patients undergoing brain or spinal surgery.
   - Specialist knowledge of neurophysiology and monitoring techniques is required.

6. Regional anaesthesia and anaesthesia for trauma :
   - Focuses on nerve blocks for specific procedures or to manage pain after surgery.
   - Useful for orthopaedic and trauma surgery.

7. Outpatient anaesthesia :
   - For operations that allow the patient to go home the same day.
   - Requires mastery of techniques that offer rapid recovery and minimise side effects.

8. Intensive care anaesthesia :
   - Anaesthetists specialise in the care of seriously ill patients in intensive care units.
   - They manage organ failure, haemodynamic imbalances and respiratory complications.

9. Anaesthesia for transplantation :
   - Management of patients undergoing organ transplants such as liver, heart or kidney.
   - In-depth knowledge of organ physiology and immunosuppression required.

10. Research in anaesthesia :
   - For those interested in academic and clinical research.
   - Topics can range from mechanisms of anaesthesia to improved techniques and drugs.

These specialities offer anaesthetists the opportunity to deepen their skills and knowledge in specific areas, ensuring that patients are optimally cared for according to their particular needs. Specialisation also enables anaesthetists to work closely with other healthcare professionals, creating an interdisciplinary approach to patient care.

Networking, mentoring and leadership in anaesthesia

Anaesthesia, like other medical specialities, is constantly evolving. To develop and progress in this field, it is essential to cultivate professional relationships, adopt a leadership role and benefit from the sound advice of mentors. Let's look at these three pillars:

1. Networking :
    Importance :
        Networking allows you to meet colleagues, share knowledge and experience and access career and research opportunities.
        It also facilitates access to resources, training and innovations in the field.
    How to do it:
        Conferences and seminars: Attend national and international anaesthesia conferences to meet experts and peers.
        Professional associations: Membership of organisations such as the Société d'Anesthésie et de Réanimation or equivalent international bodies.
        Professional social networks: Use platforms such as LinkedIn or specialist forums to exchange ideas with colleagues from all over the world.

2. Mentoring :
Importance :
A mentor provides advice, shares experiences and guides the mentee's professional development.

Mentoring helps with decision-making, navigating career challenges and acquiring advanced skills.

How to find it :
Institutional programmes: Some hospitals or academic institutions offer formal mentoring programmes.

Direct application: If you admire a professional for their expertise, don't hesitate to ask them for a mentoring role.

Discussion groups and workshops: These can be an opportunity to meet potential mentors.

3. Leadership :
Importance :
Leadership skills enable anaesthetists to lead teams, improve clinical processes and contribute to the development of the field.

A good anaesthesia leader can have a positive influence on the progress of operations, patient safety and the well-being of the team.

How to develop it :
Specific training: Taking part in programmes or seminars focusing on medical leadership.

Commitment: Active involvement in hospital committees, working groups and research projects.

Listening and communication: Cultivating these skills is essential for understanding the needs of the team and making informed decisions.

In summary, the combination of networking, mentoring and leadership is crucial for any anaesthetist wishing to excel in their career. It not only enables professional development, but also makes a significant contribution to advancing the specialty and improving patient care.

Chapter 24:
TECHNOLOGICAL INNOVATIONS IN ANAESTHESIA

The emergence of anaesthesia guided by artificial intelligence

The medical world is being turned upside down by the arrival of artificial intelligence (AI), and the field of anaesthesia is no exception. From automated systems to analytical algorithms, AI promises to revolutionise the way anaesthetic care is delivered. Let's take a look at this exciting development.

1. Historical background:
   - **Birth of medical AI**: The first steps towards the use of AI in medicine were taken in the 1960s with diagnostic assistance systems.
   - **Growing adoption**: Over the past few decades, AI has found its way into a variety of medical specialties, from radiology to cardiology, thanks to technological advances.

2. AI in anaesthesia :
   - **Automated systems** : Devices have been developed to administer anaesthetic agents based on physiological parameters, optimising the dose and reducing the risk of error.
   - **Predictive analysis**: Thanks to AI, it is now possible to analyse thousands of pieces of data in real time to anticipate possible complications during an operation.
   - **Pain management**: Algorithms can help predict a patient's response to different analgesics, enabling more precise management of postoperative pain.

3. Advantages :

   Greater accuracy: AI can process astronomical amounts of data at phenomenal speed, improving the accuracy of clinical decisions.

   Enhanced safety: AI systems can quickly identify anomalies, reducing the risk of complications.

   Time optimisation: The anaesthetist can concentrate on other aspects of patient care, by entrusting certain repetitive tasks to the AI.

4. Challenges and concerns :

   Reliability: Like any technological tool, AI is not infallible. Its dependence on correct and complete data is crucial.

   Ethics: Who is liable in the event of an AI system error? How can the confidentiality of patient data be guaranteed?

   Training: Integrating AI into anaesthesia requires specific training for professionals to ensure optimal use.

5. Future prospects :

   Personalised care: With advances in AI, it will be possible to offer even more personalised anaesthesia based on the genetic, physiological and historical profile of each patient.

   Human-machine collaboration: Rather than replacing anaesthetists, AI is positioned as an assistance tool, enabling joint and optimised decision-making.

   Research and innovation: AI opens the door to new research methods, offering unprecedented insights and facilitating the development of new anaesthetic techniques and drugs.

The integration of artificial intelligence into anaesthesia is the dawn of a new era. While recognising its immense potential, it is essential to approach this transition with caution, always placing the patient's well-being and safety at the centre of our concerns.

New systems and anaesthesia equipment

Medical technology is evolving rapidly, and the field of anaesthesia is no exception. Recent innovations in devices and equipment aim to improve patient safety, the precision of drug administration, and the comfort and efficiency of the anaesthetist's work. Here is an overview of some of the most significant advances.

1. Automated drug delivery systems :
   Intelligent pumps : These pumps can be programmed to deliver specific doses of anaesthetic at precise intervals, reducing the risk of human error.
   Real-time feedback systems: Some modern devices are capable of automatically adjusting the dose of anaesthetic according to physiological parameters such as blood pressure or oxygen saturation.
2. Advanced airway management devices :
   Video-laryngoscopes: These devices use a small camera to view the trachea, making intubation easier, especially in difficult cases.
   Supraglottic intubation masks: Improved versions of these masks offer a better seal and reduce the risk of aspiration.

3. Enhanced patient monitors :
   Multi-parametric monitors: These devices consolidate several vital measurements into a single screen, providing a complete overview of the patient's condition.

Capnography: New capnograph models offer more accurate graphics and real-time alerts to monitor patient ventilation.

4. Exhaled gas analysis systems :
   These devices measure the concentrations of various gases in the patient's exhaled air, providing information on metabolism, perfusion and ventilation.

5. Peripheral nerve stimulators :
   Used to precisely locate nerves before nerve blocks, these devices have seen an improvement in their accuracy and ease of use.

6. Augmented reality systems :
   Augmented reality glasses can guide anaesthetists during complex procedures, such as the insertion of an epidural catheter, by superimposing anatomical images on the real view.

7. Portable devices :
   Compact, portable monitors can now be used to monitor patients outside the operating theatre, for example during transport.

8. Information systems in anaesthesia :
   These digital systems centralise patient data, facilitate documentation and can even be integrated with electronic medical records to improve care coordination.

Anaesthesia technology is constantly evolving, with the aim of improving the quality and safety of care. While these innovations are promising, they require ongoing training for professionals to ensure that they are used in the safest possible way.

Telemedicine and its role in anaesthesia

Telemedicine, defined as the provision of medical services at a distance using information and communication technologies, has grown exponentially in recent years. In the field of anaesthesia, it offers unique opportunities to improve access to care, quality and efficiency. Here is an overview of its role in anaesthesia.

1. Preoperative remote assessment :
    Pre-anaesthetic consultations can be carried out via videoconference, to assess the patient's general condition, take their medical history and prepare them for the operation.
    These assessments are particularly useful for patients who live a long way from medical centres or who have difficulty travelling.

2. Post-operative follow-up :
    After surgery, telemedicine can be used to monitor patients' progress, assess their pain, adjust analgesic treatments and answer any questions or concerns they may have.

3. Training and education :
    Telemedicine platforms facilitate the ongoing training of anaesthetists, enabling real-time exchanges with experts, online seminars and even simulations.

4. Real-time assistance :
    In remote areas or where there are no specialists, an anaesthetist can guide a less experienced healthcare professional via telemedicine during a procedure, offering advice and expertise in real time.

5. Coordination with other specialists :
   Telemedicine facilitates collaboration between anaesthetists and other specialists (cardiologists, pulmonologists, etc.) for multidisciplinary care, especially for patients with complex co-morbidities.

6. Remote monitoring :
   Some equipment enables a patient's vital parameters to be transmitted in real time to a monitoring centre, where an anaesthetist can intervene if standards deviate.

7. Access to databases and decision-support tools :
   Telemedicine systems can be integrated with medical databases, providing anaesthetists with up-to-date information and decision-making tools during a procedure.

Challenges and ethical considerations :
   Telemedicine in anaesthesia, as in other specialities, raises questions about data confidentiality, the security of information transmitted and medical liability.
   It is essential that the platforms used comply with current safety standards and regulations.

Telemedicine offers considerable opportunities to improve the practice of anaesthesia, especially in underserved areas. However, its adoption requires appropriate training of professionals, a robust technological infrastructure, and clear regulations to ensure safe and effective care.

Chapter 25:
THE FUTURE OF ANAESTHESIA

Technological innovations and their impact

Anaesthesia, like many other medical fields, is constantly evolving thanks to technological innovations. These advances are transforming the way anaesthetic procedures are carried out, improving patient safety and increasing the efficiency of medical staff.

1. Advanced monitoring :

   Non-invasive devices: Innovations such as non-invasive continuous blood pressure measurement and brain oxygen saturation allow real-time monitoring without the inconvenience of invasive devices.

   Point-of-care ultrasound: Now an essential tool in anaesthesia, point-of-care ultrasound makes it easier to visualise anatomical structures, particularly when performing nerve blocks or inserting catheters.

2. Computerised anaesthesia :

   Computer-assisted anaesthesia delivery systems allow more precise delivery of anaesthetic agents, adjusting the dose in real time according to the patient's needs.

3. Anaesthesia Information Systems (AIS) :

   These systems centralise patient data, facilitate documentation, optimise billing and can be integrated with electronic medical records, improving care coordination.

4. Artificial intelligence and machine learning :
    These technologies are beginning to be integrated into anaesthesia, for example to predict risks or complications in a patient, to guide decision-making, or to optimise post-operative pain management.

5. Augmented reality and virtual reality :
    These tools can be used for training and simulation, enabling anaesthetists to practise complex procedures in a secure virtual environment.
    Virtual reality is also being studied as a means of reducing patients' pre-operative anxiety, by immersing them in soothing environments.

6. Wearables and connected objects :
    Wearable devices can monitor patients' vital signs after an operation, transmitting data in real time to healthcare professionals and enabling rapid intervention in the event of an anomaly.

7. Robotics in anaesthesia :
    Although robotics is mainly associated with surgery, robot guides or robotic assistants can also be used to carry out certain tasks in anaesthesia, such as preparing and administering medication.

Impact of innovations :
    Improved safety: Increased monitoring and more precise devices reduce the risk of errors and complications.
    Time optimisation: Automated or assisted systems free up time, allowing anaesthetists to concentrate on other aspects of care.
    Enhanced training: Simulation, virtual reality and other technological tools offer more varied and comprehensive training opportunities.

Personalised care: Data analysis tools enable us to better understand the specific needs of each patient and adjust care accordingly.

Technological innovations in anaesthesia are paving the way for safer, more effective and more personalised care. However, they require ongoing training for professionals, adaptation of protocols and constant evaluation to ensure that they are used optimally.

Research and development in anaesthesia

Research and development (R&D) plays a crucial role in the evolution and improvement of anaesthesia. While anaesthesia has come a long way since its inception, there are ongoing efforts to refine techniques, improve patient safety and optimise surgical outcomes. Here is an overview of R&D in anaesthesia.

1. New anaesthetic agents :

   Objective: To develop drugs that offer faster induction and recovery, are less toxic and have fewer side effects.

   Current progress: Studies are being carried out on agents that target specific neuronal pathways, thereby minimising side effects while ensuring adequate anaesthesia.

2. Methods of administration :

   The aim of the research is to improve the accuracy of drug administration, reduce errors and ensure consistent anaesthesia tailored to the patient.

   The use of pumps and automated devices to precisely control the delivery of anaesthetic agents is a fast-growing field.

3. Improved monitoring :
  The aim is to monitor patients more comprehensively and accurately, enabling early detection of potential complications.
  Emerging technologies, such as cerebral oxygenation monitors and portable ultrasound scanners, are being studied for their usefulness in anaesthesia.

4. Non-pharmacological techniques :
  R&D is also exploring non-drug methods of inducing anaesthesia or sedation, such as transcranial magnetic stimulation.

5. Personalised anaesthesia :
  With the advent of personalised medicine, research is being carried out to adapt anaesthesia to the patient's individual genetics and physiology.

6. Safety and quality :
  Research into medical errors, complications and preventive measures is essential to improve safety in anaesthesia.

7. Anaesthesia under special conditions :
  R&D is also looking at anaesthesia in specific situations, such as extreme emergencies, natural disasters or low-resource conditions.

8. Environmental impact :
  Some anaesthetic agents have a global warming potential. Research is aimed at developing more environmentally-friendly alternatives.

9. Interdisciplinary collaboration :
  R&D in anaesthesia is not isolated. It collaborates with other fields such as pharmacology, neurology, biotechnology, medical engineering and other specialities to develop innovative solutions.

Research and development in anaesthesia aims to constantly improve patient care. By exploring new techniques, medicines and technologies, and collaborating with other disciplines, anaesthesia continues to make progress towards safer, more effective and more personalised care for patients worldwide.

The vision of the future : the nurse anaesthetist of tomorrow

Anaesthesia, like other areas of medicine, is constantly evolving, driven by technological advances, scientific discoveries and the changing needs of society. In this trajectory of progress, the role of the nurse anaesthetist is bound to evolve and adapt. Let's take a closer look at what the nurse anaesthetist of tomorrow might look like.

1. Advanced technology integration :
   • Tomorrow's nurse anaesthetist will probably be even more comfortable with cutting-edge technologies, using tools such as artificial intelligence for patient monitoring, telemedicine for consultations, and augmented reality for continuing education.

2. Multidisciplinary expertise :
   • The increasing complexity of cases, with patients having multiple co-morbidities, will require expertise in several disciplines. Nurse anaesthetists could have advanced skills in cardiology, neurology or pharmacology, for example.

3. Patient-centred :
   • The trend towards more personalised care will continue. Tomorrow's nurse anaesthetist will be highly skilled at understanding and responding to patients' individual needs, incorporating factors such as

165

genetics, lifestyle and personal preferences into the anaesthetic plan.

4. Leader and educator :
   * In addition to direct care, the nurse anaesthetist will play a greater leadership role within medical teams, helping to develop protocols, train new generations and raise public awareness of anaesthesia-related issues.

5. Adaptability and resilience :
   * Faced with a constantly changing medical environment, the ability to adapt quickly to new situations, whether it's a pandemic, a technological advance or a new drug, will be essential.

6. Commitment to sustainability :
   * Concern for the environment and sustainability will increase. This means that the nurse anaesthetist will be involved in making choices that minimise environmental impact, whether through the choice of medicines, the use of eco-responsible equipment or the adoption of sustainable practices.

7. Ethics and humanism :
   * Despite technological advances, the human aspect of care will remain at the heart of the profession. The ability to interact with empathy, understand ethical dilemmas and defend patients' rights will be of paramount importance.

The future of the nurse anaesthetist looks promising, marked by innovation, specialisation and a profound sense of humanity. These health professionals will continue to be essential pillars of the patient's surgical journey, ensuring the safety, comfort and respect of each individual.

Chapter 26:
RESOURCES
AND ADDITIONAL REFERENCES

Reference books and key articles

Anaesthesia is a vast and constantly evolving field. In order to provide adequate training and keep up to date with the latest discoveries and techniques, it is essential to refer to reference books and articles. Here is a non-exhaustive list of the essential works in this field:

Reference books :
- **Miller's Anesthesia** by Ronald D. Miller et al.
  - A must-have for all anaesthesia professionals. This book provides comprehensive coverage of the discipline, from the fundamental basics to clinical applications.
- **Basics of Anesthesia** by Robert K. Stoelting and Ronald D. Miller.
  - A concise and clear introduction to the practice of anaesthesia, ideal for beginners or as a revision guide.
- **Clinical Anesthesia** by Paul G. Barash, Bruce F. Cullen, and Robert K. Stoelting.
  - A detailed guide to the clinical aspects of anaesthesia, highlighting the latest techniques and recommendations.
- **Morgan & Mikhail's Clinical Anesthesiology** by John F. Butterworth, David C. Mackey, and John D. Wasnick.
  - Another essential book providing a comprehensive overview of the clinical aspects of anaesthesia.

167

- **Anesthesia and Co-Existing Disease** by Robert K. Stoelting and Stephen F. Dierdorf.
  - A specialist guide to the management of patients with co-morbidities, offering anaesthetic strategies tailored to each pathology.

Key articles :

It is difficult to list specific articles as anaesthesia research is constantly being updated. However, here are a few reference journals where essential articles can be found:

- **Anesthesiology** - The official journal of the American Society of Anesthesiologists. It publishes clinical and experimental research, reviews, and educational articles.
- **British Journal of Anaesthesia** - An international journal covering all aspects of anaesthesia.
- **Anesthesia & Analgesia** - Publishes research on clinical practice, education, and policy related to anesthesia.
- **European Journal of Anaesthesiology** - Focuses on clinical and basic research in anaesthesia, intensive care and pain medicine.

Tip: Medical literature evolves rapidly, so it's essential to regularly consult medical databases such as PubMed or Medline, and to attend professional conferences to keep up to date with the latest key publications.

Reference books :

- **Précis d'anesthésie et de réanimation** by Olivier Fourcade, Bernard Geeraerts and Pierre Coriat.
  - A reference in anaesthesia and resuscitation, covering both the fundamentals and clinical applications.
- Anaesthesia and resuscitation in cardiac surgery by Gilles Gueret and Pascal Rozec.

- This book focuses on cardiac anaesthesia, a particularly specialised and complex sub-field.
- **Pharmacology in anaesthesiology** by Serge Molliex, Bruno Riou and Olivier Fourcade.
  - A guide to the drugs and agents used in anaesthesia, providing an overview of their pharmacodynamics, pharmacokinetics and side effects.
- **Emergency anaesthesia** by Yannick Le Manach, Pierre-Géraud Claret and Thomas Fuchs-Buder.
  - A book that looks at emergency situations in anaesthesia, providing protocols and recommendations.
- **Paediatric anaesthesia** by Gérard Pons and Véronique Gauthier-Moulinier.
  - This book looks at the particularities of anaesthesia in children, a discipline in its own right.

Key articles :
Research in anaesthesia is dynamic and constant. For articles, it is advisable to follow the leading French-language medical journals. Here are a few suggestions:
- **Annales Françaises d'Anesthésie et de Réanimation** - A reference journal for French-speaking anaesthetists. It publishes research, reviews and recommendations.
- **La Revue des SAMU** - Although it focuses mainly on emergency medicine, it also covers relevant topics in anaesthesia.
- **Pain: Assessment - Diagnosis - Treatment** - A specialist journal on pain management, including aspects related to anaesthesia.

Tip: As with English-language books, medical research evolves rapidly. It is therefore advisable to consult databases such as PubMed regularly (even if the articles are mainly in English, targeted searches can help you find articles in French), and to attend French-language conferences and training courses to keep up to date.

Professional organisations and conferences

Professional organisations play a vital role in continuing education, updating protocols and promoting research in anaesthesia. Here are some of the main French-speaking organisations and conferences in this field.

Professional organisations :
- **Société Française d'Anesthésie et de Réanimation (SFAR):** This is the main organisation for anaesthetists in France. It offers recommendations, training and events throughout the year.
- **Collège National des Anesthésistes Réanimateurs Libéraux (CNARL):** represents private practice anaesthetists.
- **Association des Anesthésiologistes du Québec (AAQ)**: represents anaesthesiologists in Quebec and offers continuing education programmes.
- **Société Belge d'Anesthésie et de Réanimation (SBAR):** An organisation representing anaesthetists in Belgium, which also offers training programmes.

Notable conferences :
- **SFAR Annual Congress**: This is the main event for anaesthetists in France. It offers a multitude of conferences, workshops and sessions on the latest advances in the field.
- **Journées Franco-Suisses d'Anesthésie**: An annual meeting between anaesthetists from France and Switzerland.

- **AAQ Congress**: The AAQ brings together anaesthesiologists from Quebec and elsewhere to discuss the latest advances and best practices.
- **Belgian Anaesthesia Days**: Organised by the SBAR, these days bring together professionals from Belgium and neighbouring countries.
- **Renc'AR**: An annual meeting in anaesthesia and intensive care dedicated to daily practice and innovations.

In addition to these specifically French-speaking conferences, there are many international events where English is the main language, but which are also relevant to French-speaking anaesthetists. These events, such as the congress of the European Society of Anaesthesiology, can be an excellent opportunity to exchange with colleagues from all over the world and to learn more about international advances in the field of anaesthesia.

Networking and professional communities

In the medical field, and more specifically in anaesthesia, networking and belonging to professional communities are essential. They enable professionals to exchange knowledge, share experiences, learn about the latest advances, find opportunities for continuing education and collaborate on research projects.

Why is networking important?
- **Exchanging knowledge**: Talking with colleagues allows you to learn about new techniques, new protocols and the latest advances in care and treatment.

- **Professional opportunities**: Networking can lead to job opportunities, invitations to conferences or research collaborations.
- **Professional and emotional support**: Clinical challenges can be stressful. Talking to colleagues who have been through similar experiences can offer support and different perspectives.

Where and how to network?
- **Conferences and congresses**: Attending professional conferences is one of the best ways to meet colleagues and exchange ideas.
- **Workshops and training courses**: These often provide opportunities to work in small groups and forge closer links with other professionals.
- **Online communities**: forums, Facebook groups, LinkedIn and other social platforms provide spaces for exchanging ideas, asking questions and sharing resources.
- **Professional associations and societies**: Joining a professional organisation is essential for any anaesthetist. These groups often offer valuable resources, training events and volunteering opportunities.

Notable professional communities in anaesthesia :
- **Société Française d'Anesthésie et de Réanimation (SFAR)**: In addition to its conferences, the SFAR offers workshops, working groups and online resources for its members.
- **Anaesthesia-Recovery Forum**: This is an online forum where anaesthetists can discuss clinical issues, share experiences and ask for advice.
- **Special Interest Groups**: There are many special interest groups, such as those focusing on paediatric anaesthesia, pain management or obstetric anaesthesia.

Finally, networking in anaesthesia is not only an opportunity to learn, but also to contribute. Sharing your own experiences and knowledge can help other professionals and enrich the community as a whole.